The FastDay Cookbook

Other FastDiet Books

The FastDiet
by Dr. Michael Mosley and Mimi Spencer

The FastDiet Cookbook
by Mimi Spencer with Dr. Sarah Schenker

FastExercise
by Dr. Michael Mosley with Peta Bee

The FastDay Cookbook

Delicious Low-Calorie Meals
to Enjoy While on *The FastDiet*

MIMI SPENCER

Photography by Romas Foord

ATRIA PAPERBACK

New York • London• Toronto • Sydney • New Delhi

ATRIA PAPERBACK
A Division of Simon & Schuster, Inc.
1230 Avenue of the Americas
New York, NY 10020

Copyright © 2014 by Mimi Spencer Limited
Photographs © 2014 by Romas Foord
A slightly different version of this work was previously published in Great Britain in 2014 by Short Books.

First Atria Paperback edition October 2014

ATRIA PAPERBACK and colophon are trademarks of Simon & Schuster, Inc.

For information about special discounts for bulk purchases, please contact Simon & Schuster Special Sales at 1-866-506-1949 or business@simonandschuster.com

The Simon & Schuster Speakers Bureau can bring authors to your live event. For more information or to book an event, contact the Simon & Schuster Speakers Bureau at 1-866-248-3049 or visit our website at www.simonspeakers.com.

Manufactured in the United States of America

10 9 8 7 6 5 4 3 2 1

Library of Congress Cataloging-in-Publication Data
Spencer, Mimi.
The fastday cookbook : delicious low-calorie meals to enjoy while on the fastdiet / Mimi Spencer ; photography by Romas Foord.—First Atria paperback edition.
       pages cm
     Low-calorie diet—Recipes. 2. Reducing diets—Recipes. I. Title.
     RM222.2.S674718 2014
     641.5'635—dc23
                             2014019292

ISBN 978-1-4767-7881-5
ISBN 978-1-4767-7884-6 (ebook)

For my incredible shrinking father

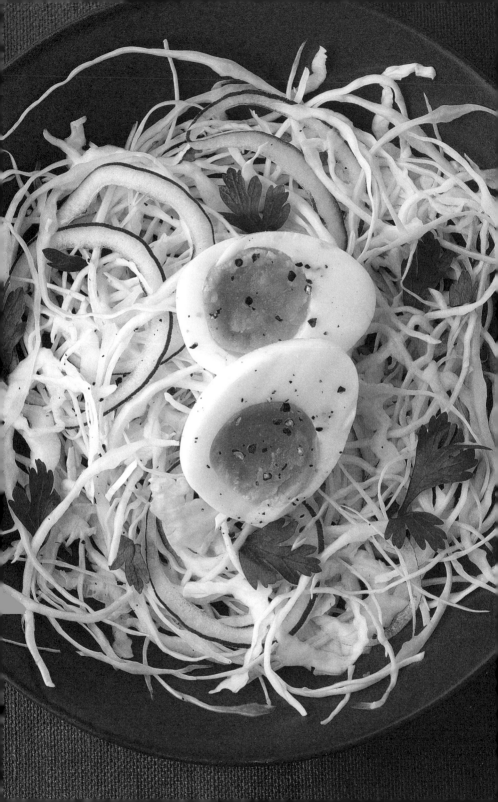

CONTENTS

INTRODUCTION

A New FastDiet Cookbook

If you happen to find yourself at the Raw Bar at the One Canada Square restaurant in London, you'll see "venison carpaccio and wild bass ceviche" on the menu, catering to "the modern carb-phobic financier." It's great to see that bankers are looking to cut back on carbs (many of them are on the FastDiet, after all). But what if you're Jo Normal? What if, instead of finding yourself at the Raw Bar, you find yourself at the fridge door? Tired and grumpy on a Fast Day, with only minutes to spare and a whole lot of hungry going on?

Well, this book is for you.

It's for people who have read *The FastDiet*, the book I coauthored with Dr. Michael Mosley, and who are keen to introduce 5:2 into their daily lives. Soon after the FastDiet took off last year, I wrote *The FastDiet Cookbook* to accompany it, a book designed to bring life, flavor, and a bit of drama to the characterless landscape of low-calorie eating. It was aimed at people who, despite wanting to lose weight, quite liked to cook on a Fast Day. But this book, *The FastDay Cookbook*, is different. FastDieters have asked me for something served straight, no twist. They've asked for simple, practical basics. They want familiar favorites and hearty food, some of it in substantial man-size portions; a decent plate of proper nosh to leave them feeling satisfied and content, even when sticking to a Fast Day calorie quota.

In short, they wanted a support system for the 5:2 diet.

So here it is. Don't expect to fall off your seat in surprise. Most of the recipes here are cherished classics, rejigged to lower the calorie content but retain every bit of flavor. I've aimed for speed and convenience, with recipes that are easy to follow rather than game-changing—chiefly because a Fast Day necessarily demotes food to fuel. That, in part, is the point. So save the dreamy recipes for other days—there'll be plenty of those.

The FastDiet: A Quick Recap

It may be radical, but the FastDiet is also wonderfully economical with its rules. All you really need to know is that:

● You eat normally for five days a week and then, for two days a week, you consume a quarter of your usual calorie intake—around 600 calories for men, 500 for women. So, it is not total "fasting," but a modified version. You won't "starve" on any given day; there are still calories coming in.

● You can do your Fast Days back to back, or split them. Michael tried both ways and found he preferred nonconsecutive days, fasting on Mondays and Thursdays. So, it is not continual fasting, but intermittent.

● Most people divide their calorie allowance between breakfast and an evening meal. You can, of course, skip breakfast and have a more substantial evening meal if it better suits your day. The key is to aim for a lengthy "fasting window" between meals.

● It does matter what you eat—plan your 500 or 600 calories by sticking, as the recipes here do, to the FastDiet mantra: "Mostly Plants and Protein." That way, you'll stay fuller longer and get adequate nutrients in your diet.

Do this, and you should experience the many benefits of Intermittent Fasting. These include:

● Weight loss of around a pound a week

● A reduction in a hormone called IGF-1, which means that you are reducing your risk of a number of age-related diseases

● The switching-on of countless repair genes

● A rest for your pancreas, boosting the effectiveness of the insulin it produces in response to elevated blood glucose. Increased insulin sensitivity will reduce your risk of obesity, diabetes, heart disease, and cognitive decline.

● A rise in the levels of neurotrophic factor in the brain, which should make you more cheerful . . . which, in a happy positive feedback, should make fasting more achievable.

What, When, and How to Eat

It's worth spending a little time preparing for a Fast Day. It matters that you have at least thought about what you're likely to eat, simply to avoid the prospect of falling face first into the nearest chocolate fudge cake the moment hunger calls.

This book contains only recipes, which would best suit an evening meal since this is the time when inspiration is usually required. Breakfast on a Fast Day—if you choose to have it—is usually a simple affair based around the humble egg. A couple of eggs, scrambled and perhaps pepped up with tarragon or chives, grainy mustard or chiles, clock in at around 200 calories and will really set you up for the day. Oatmeal—with pear and cinnamon, or berries and honey—will release energy slowly, particularly if you stick to jumbo oats. But it's supper, which requires most attention; besides, it's the thing we Fasters look forward to most during the day. It's part of what gets us through.

For many people, speed and convenience are of the essence here. Get it fast from a packet or a bag if necessary. Open a can. Poke about in the freezer. The following facts, tricks, and tips should help you meet your Fast Day target.

PROTEIN: The body does not store protein, so we recommend that you boost the protein content of your diet on Fast Days, making it a greater proportion of your daily diet on just those days. That way, you benefit from its satiating effects (protein really does make you feel fuller for longer than carbs) and you will have adequate levels of protein at all times.

MEAT: Cooking meat and poultry with its skin on will maximize its flavor and prevent it from drying out, but don't eat the skin—it's a calorie trap. Also, roast or grill meat on a rack over a baking pan to allow excess fat to drip away. A grill pan will channel fat into the grooves and away from your plate.

EGGS: A great start to a Fast Day, full of healthy fats, protein (all 9 essential amino acids), B vitamins, and minerals. People who consume egg protein for breakfast are more likely to feel full during the day than those whose breakfasts contain wheat protein.

VEGETABLE PROTEIN: Rather than rely solely on animal proteins, try to include vegetable protein on a Fast Day when you can. It's generally cheaper (and better for the planet, too). Include nuts, mushrooms, tofu, and legumes of all kinds. Legumes, such as lentils, chickpeas, split peas, and beans are excellent sources of plant protein and fiber, and rank low on the GI (glycemic index) scale.

PLANTS: Favor leafy greens over starchy vegetables. Steam, boil, blanch, and grill; don't overcook and don't fry. Roasting vegetables in a hot oven will caramelize their natural sugars; lightly spray with olive oil to stop them from drying out.

DAIRY: Use low-fat crème fraîche or low-fat plain yogurt. Avoid butter on a Fast Day—it racks up the calories. Certain cheeses are lower in calories than others: feta, for example, is made from sheep's milk and is a good source of protein, calcium, and vitamin B12. Low-fat mozzarella is a handy staple in the fridge. Choose sharp cheese instead of mild—its stronger flavor means you need less of it.

OILS AND FATS: I use cooking spray when I can—in general, most oil sprays provide about 15 calories per two-second spray. Otherwise, use olive oil, but sparingly. You only need expensive extra-virgin olive oil for salad dressings and drizzling; use standard olive oil for cooking. It's possible to avoid oil entirely when sautéing onion: Simply use a nonstick pan and a splash of water instead of oil, and watch that it doesn't stick. Alternatively, use a silicone brush to apply oil to a pan and dab away any excess with paper towels. Most oils contain around 120 calories per tablespoon, so it's worth being particular about it when cooking.

CARBS: On a Fast Day? Not so much. The ones to avoid entirely are the fast-release blood-sugar spikers. Tropical fruits and juices are off-menu. As are white carbs. Slow-release carbohydrates—such as the jumbo oats in a bowl of oatmeal, or brown basmati rice—will, however, help fill you up and keep you going. If you find that a plate is naked without a carb fix, try shirataki noodles. Made of a water-soluble fiber called glucomannan, they have no fat, sugar, gluten, or starch. What you'll need to add, though, is flavor.

Fast Day Flavor . . . Without Fat

The recipes in this book are designed to add big bolts of flavor wherever possible. Here's how:

SPICE IT: Herbs and spices should feature heavily in Fast Day cooking. Cumin seeds, cardamom pods, paprika, basil, cilantro . . . they are central to a dish when fats are scarce. As a rule, use fresh herbs over dried as they tend to have greater flavor and more nutrients.

SPIKE IT: With mustard, onions, shallots, vinegar, chiles . . . anything that brings your fork to attention. There's much to be said, for instance, for the sweet joy of roast garlic: Bake a whole head of it, sealed in foil with a splash of water, for 40 minutes. Once cooled, squeeze out the pulp and add to . . . anything at all. Green beans would be a good place to start. You may also like to embrace the Fantastic Five—lime juice, soy sauce, fresh ginger, garlic, and Thai fish sauce—a combination known as *nam jim* which delivers a hit of flavor for very few calories.

BOOST IT: Use sun-dried tomatoes or porcini mushrooms in place of bacon or chorizo: both ingredients lend a smoky depth to a dish without the addition of careless calories. Paprika will perform the same flavor favor. To-mato paste will up the ante in any tomato-based recipe (as will the merest pinch of sugar). Anchovies and capers will give a useful savory, salty bite. And remember, when the world gives you lemons . . . make a salad dress-ing. Sometimes just a squeeze of lemon is enough to jazz up a plate.

The Fast Day Kitchen: What To Have On Hand

Get in the habit of having Fast-friendly food around—just enough to allow you to grab a quick meal when you're fasting and famished. Just enough to stop you from dialing out for pizza.

IN THE FRIDGE
Eggs
Smoked salmon
Low-fat hummus, low-fat yogurt, and low-fat crème fraîche
Feta, cottage cheese, and low-fat mozzarella
Scallions
Chiles
Fresh herbs
Nonstarchy veggies: cauliflower, broccoli, peppers, radishes,
     cherry tomatoes, celery, cucumber, mushrooms, lettuce, sugar
     snaps, salad leaves, and a bag of baby spinach
Carrots
Lemons
Strawberries, blueberries, and apples

IN THE CUPBOARD
Cans of tuna in spring water
Cans of beans—such as cannellini, cranberry beans,
     and chickpeas

Tomato paste

Garlic

Onions—red and white

Mustard—Dijon and yellow mustard

Vinegar—balsamic and white wine; try balsamic vinegar in a
spritzer for salad

Olive oil

Cooking spray

Spices, including cumin and coriander

Red pepper flakes

Nuts—unsalted are preferable; eat with caution as they are
generally high in calories

Pickles—guindilla, jalapeños, cornichons, capers

Bouillon cubes, miso paste

Sea salt and freshly ground black pepper

Unsweetened muesli

Sugar-free jelly

Shirataki noodles

IN THE FREEZER

Root ginger—it is best grated from frozen

Stock—in empty (clean) soup and milk cartons

Soup—homemade or store-bought, in single portions

Blueberries (strawberries don't freeze well)

Peas

How the Book Works

Each calorie count is for a single portion, even if the recipe produces
enough for 2 or 4 (or more) people. Recipes which produce larger quantities will generally be ideal for freezing. At the end of the book, you'll find a
calorie-counted index to help you choose a dish that fits your calorie quota
on any given day.

Where appropriate, recipes have "serve with" options, and "goes well
with" suggestions from elsewhere in the book. Add the calories together
to get your total for the meal. Most of the dishes are ideal for nonfasting

family members too—simply add potatoes, rice, or bread to make a more substantial plate.

A Few Words of Fast Day Wisdom

Much has been written, and many stories shared, about the FastDiet and how to succeed with the 5:2 approach. You'll find plenty of advice and tips on www.thefastdiet.co.uk. Here's my distilled version. A 5:2 bouillon cube, if you like:

● Drink plenty of water. Get into the habit of drinking a glass of water before and after Fast Day meals. And drink water when you feel hungry, too (it really does help; the stomach is a simple beast). Supplement your water intake with herbal tea, black coffee, miso soup—but not juice, which can rack up the sugars. Diet Coke? OK, if it's the only thing that gets you through.

● Remember, your aim is to secure a food-free breathing space for your body. So snack with caution: all calories count on a Fast Day, and your objective is to achieve as long a fasting window as possible. If you must snack, have berries, an apple, a carrot. Not a bag of chips.

● In any one week, work out a pattern that suits you: Fast on a day when you are busy but not overly social; have breakfast as part of your calorie budget if that works for you—skip it if not. For lots more advice and personal takes, go to www.thefastdiet.co.uk.

● Get a handle on hunger: the pangs will pass. We often eat because we're bored or emotional rather than actually hungry. Try to differentiate between the two. Real hunger won't hurt you—not for the mere handful of hours until you get your next food fix.

● Stay calm. Going to 510 calories (or 615 for a man) won't obliterate a fast. While there's no particular "magic" to 500 or 600 calories, do try to stick broadly to these numbers; you do need clear parameters to make the strategy effective in the medium term.

● Stay positive. Don't be disheartened if you "plateau" and don't lose weight in any given week; look at the medium term and remember the health benefits beyond weight loss—the real dividend is its long-term health gains, the prospect of cutting your risk of a range of diseases, including diabetes, heart disease, and some cancers. There is also evidence that it will slow the aging process and benefit your brain.

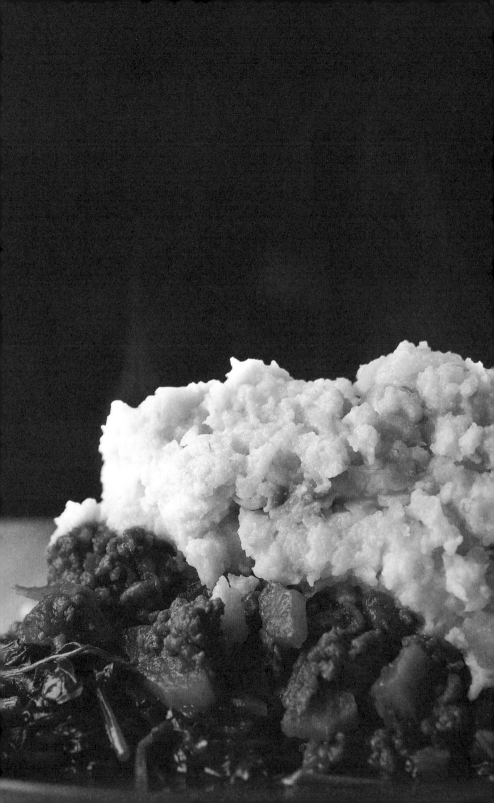

Fast Day Favorites

The Classics. Only Skinnier.

We're all comforted by dishes we know and love, recipes we recognize, and food that makes us nod in understanding, appreciation, and anticipation. Then there are the world-class classics: coq au vin, Thai curry, chili con carne, spaghetti. . . . Most of us eat them day in day out, but these dishes can often clock up reckless calories. Here, then, I've taken a few of our favorites and slimmed them down to better suit a Fast Day. Fats, sugars, and fast-release carbs are limited, while plants and proteins have the starring roles. You'll still find food you know, food you love. Just a darn sight skinnier.

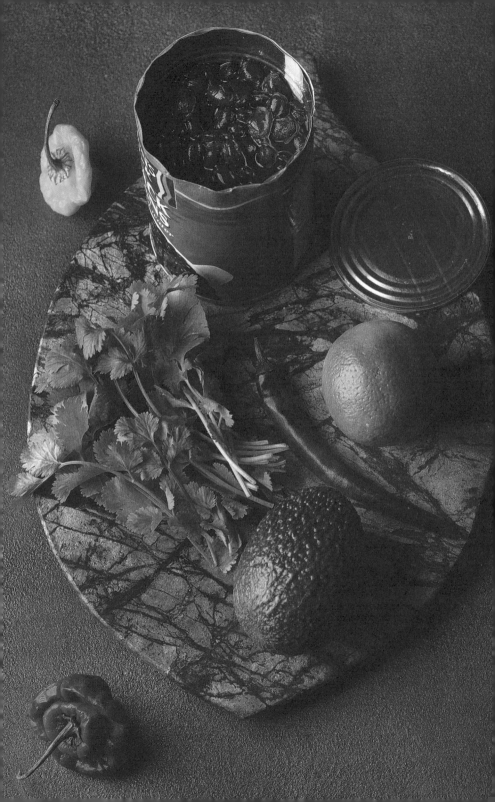

CHILI THREE WAYS . . .

. . . Mexican black bean chili

144 CALORIES PER PORTION

Serves 4

1 medium onion, finely chopped
2 medium zucchini, chopped
2 medium red bell peppers,
  seeded and finely chopped
1 medium carrot, peeled and
  finely chopped
1 medium celery stalk, chopped
1 garlic clove, crushed
1 red chile, finely chopped
  (seeded to taste)
½ teaspoon ground coriander
½ teaspoon ground cumin

1 (14-ounce/400g) can diced
  tomatoes
1 tablespoon tomato paste
1 (14-ounce/400g) can black
  beans, rinsed and drained
3½ ounces/100g frozen corn
⅓ cup/75ml water
1 tablespoon lime juice
Salt and freshly ground black
  pepper
Cilantro leaves and low-fat plain
  yogurt, for serving

Heat the oil in a large heavy-bottomed pan. Sauté the onion, zucchini, bell peppers, carrot, and celery on medium heat for 5 minutes, until softened. Add the garlic, chile, and spices, stir and cook for another 3 minutes. Stir in the tomatoes, tomato paste, beans, corn, and water and simmer for 20 to 25 minutes, until the sauce thickens. Stir in the lime juice, season, and serve with cilantro and a spoonful of yogurt.

OPTIONAL EXTRA: Serve with 1 avocado, chopped, and dressed with lemon juice (+75 calories per quarter).

... white chili with turkey

302 CALORIES PER PORTION

Serves 4

Using turkey instead of the more traditional beef will slash your calorie intake at a stroke, and give your mouth something new to try (use 93% lean turkey, which has just enough fat to keep the chili from being dry). The cannellini beans make the perfect match—full of protein, full of fiber, a Fast Day staple.

1 small onion, chopped
1 small green bell pepper,
   seeded and chopped
3 garlic cloves, thinly sliced
¾ teaspoon ancho chile powder
1 pound/450g ground turkey
   (93% lean)

1 (14-ounce/400g) can cannellini
   beans, drained and rinsed
¼ cup/60ml water
¾ teaspoon salt
¼ cup chopped cilantro
1 tablespoon lime juice

In a large skillet, heat the oil over medium heat. Add the onion, bell pepper, and garlic and cook, stirring occasionally, until tender, about 7 minutes. Stir in the chile powder and cook for 1 minute. Add the turkey and cook, breaking up lumps with a wooden spoon until the turkey is no longer pink, about 4 minutes.

Add the beans, water, and salt and cook until the beans are heated through, about 2 minutes. Stir in the cilantro and lime juice and serve.

● Ancho chile powder is smoky and hot, but not killer hot. If you prefer, you can swap in your favorite chili powder, but check the label for added ingredients such as salt and other spices.

● You can add other vegetables to the chili when cooking the onion and bell pepper. Carrots or red bell peppers swapped in for the green will give sweetness. Zucchini or yellow squash will make the chili creamier.

● Feel free to swap in your favorite beans. And, if you happen to have some chicken stock around, you can use it instead of the water.

...low-cal chili con carne

241 CALORIES PER PORTION

Serves 4

1 pound/450g lean ground beef
Cooking spray
2 medium onions, diced
2 garlic cloves, crushed
1 medium red bell pepper,
  seeded and diced
1 teaspoon chili powder, or to
  taste
½ teaspoon crushed red pepper
  flakes
1 teaspoon ground cumin
1 bay leaf

9 ounces/250g mushrooms, sliced
1 (14-ounce/400g) can diced
  tomatoes
2 tablespoons tomato paste
Pinch of sugar
Scant 1 cup/200ml beef stock
  or boiling water with a beef
  bouillon cube
1 (14-ounce/400g) can kidney
  beans, rinsed and drained
Salt and freshly ground black
  pepper

Sauté the beef in a large frying pan until browned and set aside. Heat the oil and sauté the onion, garlic, and bell pepper for 3 to 4 minutes, until softened. Add the spices, bay leaf, mushrooms, tomatoes, tomato paste, and sugar and cook for another 3 to 4 minutes. Add the browned meat and stock to the pan and simmer for 15 minutes. Add the beans and cook for 30 minutes—longer if possible to enrich the chili. Season and serve.

Traditionally, of course, chili tends to demand carbs on the side. But on a Fast Day, avoid rice, tortillas, or potatoes and serve instead with:

● steamed kale, spinach, broccoli, sugar snaps, or finely sliced cabbage (+25 to 35 calories per 3½ ounces/100g)

● roasted butternut squash, zucchini, or Bermuda onion wedges (+20 calories per 3½ ounces/100g)

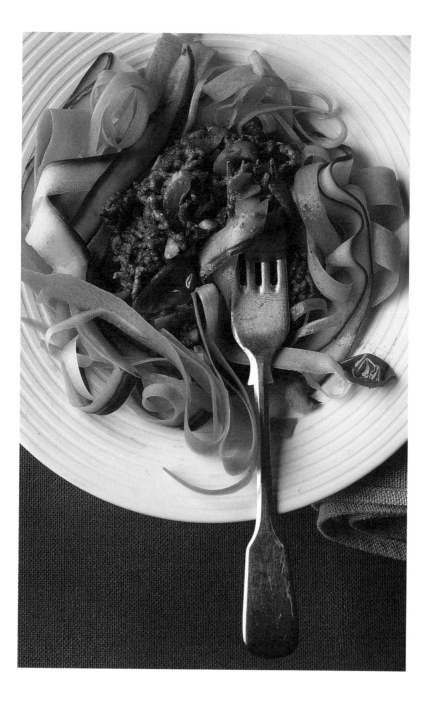

SKINNY SPAGHETTI BOLOGNESE

180 CALORIES PER PORTION

Serves 4

A family classic, but here I've lowered the GI count and raised the fiber by bumping up the vegetables. My father always adds mixed spice to his Bolognese sauce, and I'd recommend its addition for an authentic Italian touch.

Cooking spray
14 ounces/400g lean
  ground beef
1 large onion, diced
1 garlic clove, crushed
1 medium celery stalk, diced
1 medium red bell pepper,
  diced
7 ounces/200g mushrooms,
  chopped
½ teaspoon dried mixed herbs

1 teaspoon mixed spice (cumin,
  coriander, nutmeg)
1 (14-ounce/400g) can diced
  tomatoes
3 tablespoons tomato paste
1 medium zucchini, diced
Scant 1 cup/200ml beef stock
  or boiling water with a beef
  bouillon cube
Salt and freshly ground black
  pepper

Spray a large pan with a little oil, then sauté the meat until browned and set aside in a bowl. This is an important stage as the sugars from the meat will lend your Bolognese color and flavor. Add the onion, garlic, celery, and bell pepper to the pan and cook gently for 2 to 3 minutes, until softened. Add the mushrooms, herbs, mixed spice, tomatoes, and tomato paste and cook for another 3 minutes. Add the browned meat and zucchini together with the stock. Cover and simmer, stirring occasionally, for 30 minutes—longer if possible to enrich the sauce. Check the seasoning and serve.

Instead of pasta, serve with:

● steamed broccoli and cauliflower florets (+30 to 35 calories per 3½ ounces/100g)

● veggie "noodles"—stir-fried ribbons of zucchini, carrot, and leek (+35 calories per 3½ ounces/100g)

BEAN BOLOGNESE

180 CALORIES PER PORTION

Serves 2

A vegan alternative to the classic spaghetti Bolognese—high in fiber, low in fat, and full of good things.

Cooking spray
2 garlic cloves, crushed
1 medium onion, chopped
1 medium red bell pepper, seeded and diced
3½ ounces/100g button mushrooms, sliced
1 teaspoon dried mixed herbs

1 (14-ounce/400g) can diced tomatoes
1 tablespoon tomato paste
Pinch of sugar
1 (14-ounce/400g) can pinto beans, drained and rinsed
Salt and freshly ground black pepper

Coat a large nonstick skillet with some cooking spray and sauté the garlic, onion, and bell pepper for 3 minutes, until softened. Add the mushrooms, herbs, tomatoes, tomato paste, and sugar and cook for another 3 minutes. Add the beans, then cover and simmer for 20 to 30 minutes, until the sauce has slightly reduced. Season and serve.

OPTIONAL EXTRAS: Add a handful of chopped black olives (+40 calories) and garnish with torn basil leaves.

CHIPOTLE-GLAZED INDIVIDUAL MEAT LOAVES

287 CALORIES PER PORTION

Serves 4

It's a staple in every home—but meat loaf can be heavy on the calories. Here, I've made it in individual little loaves: the ultimate in portion control!

1 cup finely chopped red onion (1 medium)	¼ cup/55g no-salt-added tomato paste
½ cup finely chopped or grated carrots	2 teaspoons balsamic vinegar
3 tablespoons water	½ teaspoon chipotle powder
10 ounces/285g cremini mushrooms, finely diced	⅔ cup/60g quick-cooking oatmeal
3 garlic cloves, minced	¾ teaspoon ground fennel
	8 ounces/225g lean ground beef
1 teaspoon salt	8 ounces/225g lean ground turkey
	1 large egg

Coat a large nonstick skillet with cooking spray and heat over medium heat. Add the onion, cover, and cook, stirring often, until the onion is softened and just beginning to brown, 4 to 5 minutes. Add the carrots and 2 tablespoons of the water to the pan. Cover and cook for 2 minutes. Add the mushrooms, garlic, and salt. Cover and cook for 2 minutes. Uncover and cook, stirring occasionally to help steam escape, until the vegetables are very tender and the mixture looks dry, about 10 minutes. Transfer the sautéed vegetables to a bowl to cool to almost room temperature. Preheat the oven to 350°F. Line a baking sheet with parchment paper or a silicone baking mat. In a small bowl, stir together the tomato paste, vinegar, and chipotle powder. Measure out 2 tablespoons, transfer to another small bowl, and stir in the remaining 1 tablespoon water to loosen the mixture. Set aside to use as a glaze. Stir the remaining chipotle mixture, oatmeal, and fennel into the vegetables. Add the beef, turkey, and egg and mix until well combined (but do not overwork or the meat will toughen). Divide the meat mixture into four equal portions and shape each into a football shaped loaf on the baking sheet. (The loaves are about 4½ inches long by 2½ inches wide.)

Bake for 30 minutes. Brush with the chipotle glaze and bake until the loaves are firm, 15 minutes longer. Let the loaves stand 10 minutes before serving. Serve the meat loaf warm, at room temperature, or chilled.

FAST DAY TIP: A good way to get the mushrooms very finely diced is to quarter them and then pulse them on and off in a food processor. And as long as you have the food processor out, you can use it to finely chop the carrots, too.

OPTIONAL EXTRA: Goes well with Lemon-Pepper Broccoli with Coconut Oil, page 113 (+64 calories per portion) and thick-sliced tomato.

COQ AU VIN

239 CALORIES PER PORTION

Serves 4

A French institution, made lighter here with the merest hint of oil, just enough pancetta for flavor, and less than half a bottle of white wine. And it still tastes heavenly, promise.

Cooking spray

4 skinless, bone-in chicken thighs (about 7¾ ounces/220g each)

1¾ ounces/50g pancetta, diced

2 medium carrots, peeled and diced

2 medium onions, diced

2 medium celery stalks, diced

2 garlic cloves, crushed

2 tablespoons all-purpose flour

1¼ cups/300ml dry white wine

1¼ cups/300ml chicken stock

Small bunch of fresh tarragon, leaves chopped

Small bunch of fresh thyme, leaves picked and chopped

1 sprig fresh rosemary

9 ounces/250g small white mushrooms, halved

Salt and freshly ground black pepper

Heat a large ovenproof casserole dish and coat with the cooking spray. Season the chicken and brown on all sides until golden. Remove from the pan and set aside. Add the pancetta to the pan and cook for 2 minutes, until it releases its flavor and is browned. Add the carrots, onions, celery, and garlic and cook for 2 minutes. Add the flour, stir well, and cook for 1 minute, then add the wine and stock, scraping the base of the pan to collect the sticky bits. Return the chicken to the pan, and add the herbs. Cover and simmer for 1 hour. Add the mushrooms and cook for another 30 minutes with the lid off. Season and serve.

OPTIONAL EXTRA: Instead of regular mushrooms, use a mix of wild mushrooms, shiitake, oyster, or chanterelles.

● Goes well with a Boston lettuce salad plus Fast Day Dressing (page 143).

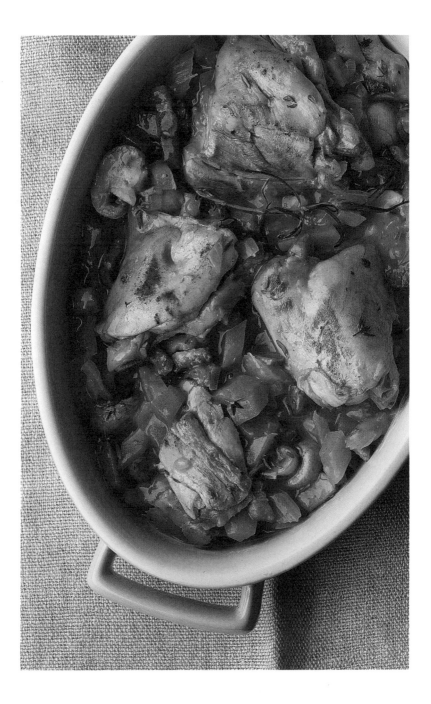

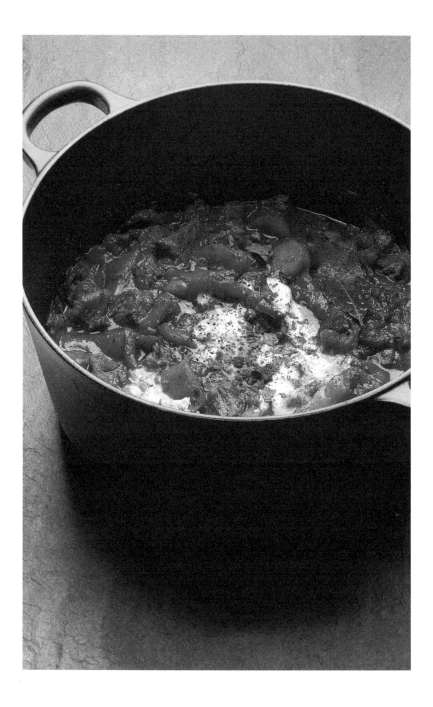

HOT PAPRIKA GOULASH

275 CALORIES PER PORTION

Serves 4

1¼ pounds/565g stewing beef, trimmed of fat and cubed
Cracked black pepper
Cooking spray
2 medium onions, sliced
2 garlic cloves, crushed
1 tablespoon sweet paprika
2 teaspoons Hungarian smoked paprika
1¾ cups/400ml beef stock or boiling water with a beef bouillon cube
1 (14-ounce/400g) can diced tomatoes
2 tablespoons tomato paste
½ teaspoon sugar
2 teaspoons apple cider vinegar
2 bay leaves
1 medium red bell pepper, seeded and coarsely chopped
1 medium yellow bell pepper, seeded and coarsely chopped
3 medium carrots, peeled and cut into chunks
Salt and freshly ground black pepper
2 tablespoons low-fat plain yogurt and chopped fresh parsley, for serving

Preheat the oven to 350°F. Season the beef with plenty of black pepper. Heat a large ovenproof, lidded casserole and coat with cooking spray. Sauté the beef until browned, remove the meat and set aside, then add the onions to the pan. Cook for 5 minutes until the onions start to soften, adding a tablespoon of stock if they are sticking. Then add the garlic and cook for another minute, stirring well. Return the beef to the pan, add the paprikas, the stock, together with the tomatoes, tomato paste, sugar, vinegar, and bay leaves. Season and bring to a simmer. Cover and transfer to the oven for 1½ hours, then add the bell peppers and carrots. Stir and return to the oven for another hour until the beef is gloriously tender. Serve with a swirl of yogurt and a generous handful of parsley.

● Goes well with Spiced Red Cabbage with Apples, page 115 (+79 calories per portion).

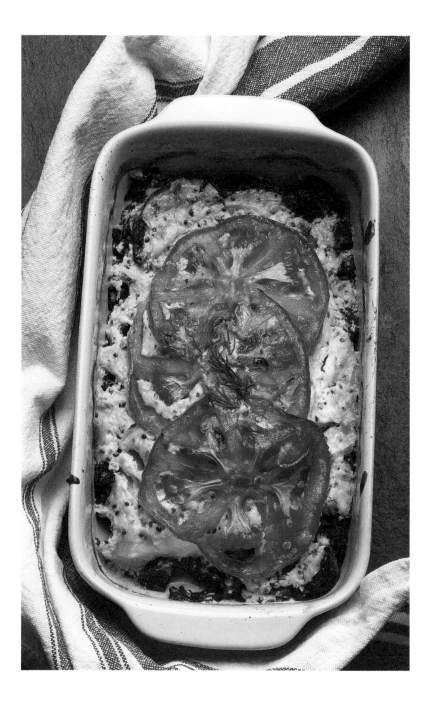

SMOKED SALMON GRATIN

276 CALORIES PER PORTION

Serves 4

1 (9-ounce/250g) bag baby spinach leaves	Salt and freshly ground black pepper
1 tablespoon grainy Dijon mustard	Zest of 1 lemon
1 heaping cup/250g low-fat crème fraîche	4 smoked salmon portions, about 5 ounces/150g each
1¾ ounces/50g sharp cheddar cheese, grated	1 beefsteak tomato, sliced
	Flat-leaf or curly parsley or dill, chopped, for serving

Preheat the oven to 350°F. Pierce the spinach bag and microwave on full power for 90 seconds. Remove the spinach from the bag and squeeze out as much moisture as possible (press it between paper towels) before transferring to an ovenproof dish. Combine the mustard, crème fraîche, cheese, and lemon zest; season carefully (the fish and the cheese will be salty). Place the fish over the drained spinach and spoon the crème fraîche mixture on top. Top with tomato slices and bake for 30 minutes. Serve with freshly chopped parsley or dill.

OPTIONAL EXTRA: Add 3½ ounces/100g cooked peeled shrimp beneath the crème fraîche mixture (+89 calories).

TANDOORI CHICKEN WITH MINT DIP AND SAAG ON THE SIDE

279 CALORIES PER PORTION

Serves 4

Ditch the heavy sauces and the mound of rice (have spiced spinach instead), and you can have a curry for under 300 calories.

For the chicken
1 heaping cup/250g low-fat
   plain yogurt
2 tablespoons tandoori spice mix
Juice of 1 lemon
Salt and pepper
8 skinless chicken drumsticks
   (about 4¼ ounces/125g each)

For the dip
3 tablespoons low-fat plain
   yogurt
Handful of fresh mint leaves
1 green chile, finely sliced
   (seeded to taste)
Salt and freshly ground black
   pepper

For the saag on the side
Cooking spray
1 medium onion, diced
2 garlic cloves, crushed
¾-inch/2cm piece fresh ginger,
   grated
½ teaspoon ground coriander
½ teaspoon ground turmeric
½ teaspoon cayenne pepper
½ teaspoon garam masala
2 cardamom pods
2 medium ripe tomatoes, cored
   and diced
1 pound/450g spinach, stems
   removed, chopped
Salt and freshly ground black
   pepper

Combine the yogurt, spice mix, lemon juice, salt, and pepper in a bowl to make a marinade. Score the chicken and add to the bowl. Mix well. Cover with plastic wrap and chill in the fridge for an hour, or overnight if possible. Preheat the oven to 400°F. Place the chicken on a wire rack over a roasting pan and bake for 20 minutes, or until it is cooked through, turning after 10 minutes. Meanwhile, for the saag, heat a large pan, spray with oil and sauté the onion over medium heat for 5 minutes. Add the garlic and cook for another 2 minutes. Add the ginger, spices, and tomatoes and cook for 2 minutes. Add the spinach in handfuls and cook until it wilts. Remove from the heat and season. Combine the dip ingredients in a small bowl and serve with the hot drumsticks and a side of the spiced saag.

BASIC BOEUF BOURGUIGNON

294 CALORIES PER PORTION

Serves 4

1 tablespoon vegetable oil
1¼ pounds/565g stewing beef, trimmed of fat and cut into cubes
9 ounces/250g shallots, peeled (pour boiling water over them to release the skins)
1 medium onion, sliced
2 tablespoons all-purpose flour
Salt and freshly ground black pepper
2 cups/500ml red wine

1¾ cups/400ml vegetable or chicken stock
3 garlic cloves, crushed
1 bouquet garni
1 cinnamon stick
2 large mushrooms, cut into quarters
2 large carrots, peeled and coarsely chopped
Chopped fresh parsley, for serving

Preheat the oven to 325°F. Heat the oil in a large, lidded ovenproof casserole and sear the beef until lightly browned on all sides. Remove from the pan and set aside. Add the shallots to the same pan, sauté for 3 to 5 minutes, or until nicely browned on all sides. Remove from the pan and set aside. Sauté the onion in the same pan, add a tablespoon of stock if it is sticking. Return the beef to the pan and sprinkle in the flour, stirring as you go. Cook for another 2 minutes, stirring all the time. Season. Gradually add the wine and stock, the garlic, bouquet garni, and cinnamon stick. Stir well to incorporate the stickiness at the base of the pan, cover tightly, and place in the oven for 2 hours. Add the browned shallots, mushrooms, and carrots and return to the oven and cook, lid on, for another 45 minutes. Serve scattered with parsley.

● Goes well with steamed green beans. Perhaps add a touch of finely chopped garlic to them for a Gallic flourish.

SUPER-FAST THAI GREEN CHICKEN CURRY

331 CALORIES PER PORTION

Serves 2

Yes, this is a chicken curry—but for a Fast Day, the meat should play second fiddle to a proper medley of vegetables. Use whatever you have on hand, and whatever you fancy today: pea eggplant, young zucchini, baby corn, snow peas, broccoli florets, bok choy, thinly sliced peppers, green beans, shiitake or oyster mushrooms, bean sprouts, frozen baby peas, or spinach. . . . Just don't overcook the veggies—they need to retain a bit of bite.

1¾ cups/400ml low-fat coconut milk
1 tablespoon Thai green curry paste
Scant ½ cup/100ml chicken stock
1 tablespoon lime juice
1 tablespoon Thai fish sauce

7 ounces/200g chicken breast, cut into strips
7 ounces/200g vegetables
1 green chile, finely sliced
Handful of fresh cilantro leaves
Lime wedges, for serving

Heat 1 tablespoon of the coconut milk in a pan, stir in the curry paste, and cook for 2 minutes to release the flavor and aroma of the paste. Add the remaining coconut milk, the stock, lime juice, and fish sauce. Bring to a simmer and cook for 10 minutes. Add the chicken and vegetables of your choice, and continue to simmer until the chicken is cooked through, about 5 minutes. Top with fresh chile and cilantro leaves, and serve with a wedge of lime.

● Try this with shrimp, tofu, or salmon instead of chicken—these will all require slightly less cooking time, 3 to 4 minutes.

● Goes well with zero-calorie shirataki noodles.

FAST DAY BIRYANI

337 CALORIES PER PORTION

Serves 4

7 ounces/200g basmati rice, rinsed

½ teaspoon saffron strands

2 garlic cloves, smashed

2 cardamom pods, smashed

1¾ cups/400ml cold water

1 tablespoon vegetable oil

1 medium onion, finely sliced

2 garlic cloves, crushed

1 teaspoon black mustard seeds

14 ounces/400g chicken tenders

Salt and freshly ground black pepper

1 teaspoon ground cumin

Put the rice, saffron, garlic, and cardamom in a saucepan with the cold water. Bring to a boil, then reduce the heat to low, cover, and cook for 10 minutes, or until all the water has been absorbed; once cooked, leave the lid on. Heat the oil in another pan, add the onion, garlic, and mustard seeds and sauté until the onion and garlic start to soften, 3 to 4 minutes. Season the chicken with salt, pepper, and ground cumin, then sauté in the same pan for a minute so that the chicken picks up some color. Cover with a lid and cook for another 3 to 4 minutes, or until the chicken is cooked through. Combine with the cooked rice, check the seasoning, and serve.

COTTAGE PIE

340 CALORIES PER PORTION

Serves 2

1 teaspoon olive oil
10½ ounces/300g extra-lean ground beef
1 large onion, diced
2 medium celery stalks, finely chopped
2 medium carrots, peeled and diced
1 (14-ounce/400g) can diced tomatoes
2 tablespoons tomato paste
1 tablespoon Worcestershire sauce

1 bay leaf
1 teaspoon chopped fresh thyme leaves
Salt and freshly ground black pepper
1¼ cups/300ml boiling water
2 beef bouillon cubes
1 pound/450g celery root, peeled and cubed
½ cup/100g low-fat crème fraîche
1 teaspoon vegetable oil
2 young leeks, trimmed and sliced (thick-coin width)

Preheat the oven to 400°F. Heat the olive oil in a large pan and brown the ground beef. Add the onion, celery, and carrots and cook for 10 minutes, until softened. Stir in the tomatoes, tomato paste, Worcestershire sauce, bay leaf, thyme, salt, pepper, water, and bouillon cubes. Bring to a boil, cover, and simmer for 30 minutes, stirring occasionally. Boil the celery root until very tender, drain, and mash with the crème fraîche until smooth. Heat the vegetable oil in a pan and sauté the leeks, then add them to the celery root mash. Pour the beef mixture into a shallow ovenproof dish and top with the celery root mash. Bake for 20 to 30 minutes, or until the top is golden brown. Serve with plenty of green leafy vegetables or steamed broccoli.

● Swap celery root mash for a mix of carrot, parsnip, or sweet potato or a combination of the three.

● Add mushrooms, chopped leeks, and lentils to bump up the meat mix— or add a layer of peas.

FAST DAY TIP: Make this in individual ramekins to control portion size; it also cooks more quickly and will freeze well in the ramekin.

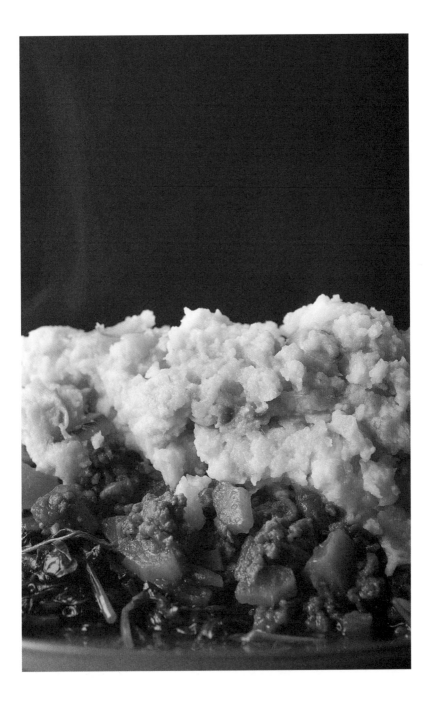

MOUSSAKA

390 CALORIES PER PORTION

Serves 4

2 teaspoons olive oil
1 medium onion, sliced
2 medium red or orange bell
  peppers, seeded and sliced
3 garlic cloves, crushed
7 ounces/200g lean ground lamb
3½ ounces/100g red lentils
1 teaspoon dried oregano, or
  2 teaspoons fresh
1 teaspoon ground allspice
2 cups/450g canned crushed
  tomatoes
1 tablespoon tomato paste

Pinch of sugar
Salt and freshly ground black
  pepper
1 medium eggplant, sliced into
  ½-inch/1cm rounds
4 medium tomatoes, sliced
2 tablespoons/25g Parmesan
  cheese, grated, plus extra for
  serving
1 cup/200g low-fat crème fraîche
1 large egg, beaten
Freshly grated nutmeg

Heat 1 teaspoon of the oil in a large pan and sauté the onion and bell peppers for 5 to 7 minutes—adding a dash of water if necessary to stop them from sticking. Add the garlic and cook for another minute, then add the lamb, and cook until it starts to brown. Add the lentils, oregano, allspice, crushed tomatoes, tomato paste, sugar, and a splash of water. Season and simmer for 15 to 20 minutes, or until the lentils are tender, adding more water if you need to. Heat the grill, place the eggplant and tomatoes on a foil-lined or nonstick baking sheet. Brush with the remaining 1 teaspoon olive oil, season, then grill for 4 minutes on each side, until slightly blackened. Combine the Parmesan, crème fraîche, egg, salt, and pepper. Spoon the meat mixture into an ovenproof dish and top with the eggplant and tomato. Add the crème fraîche mix and sprinkle with nutmeg and a little extra Parmesan. Place under a hot grill for 3 minutes, until it starts to brown and bubble. Serve with a simple green salad.

CHEAT'S TIP: Use frozen sliced peppers and canned lentils to save on prep time (one 14-ounce/400g can, drained).

ROAST BEEF HASH WITH EGGS

293 CALORIES PER PORTION

Serves 4

An all-American classic—but how to get that calorie count down? Here, I've swapped out the usual potatoes for zucchini, and bumped up the vegetables again by adding asparagus to the mix. This means your hash stays fresh and vibrant, but as delicious as any you've tried before. . . . If you want to make this dish to serve just one, cook up the mixture, divide it into four equal portions and refrigerate. When ready to make the dish, gently reheat the mixture in a small skillet and cook the egg on top as directed, then sprinkle with a tablespoon of fresh Parmesan.

1 teaspoon extra-virgin olive oil
1 large red onion, chopped
3 garlic cloves, minced
2 tablespoons water
1 pound/450g asparagus, cut into ½-inch/1cm pieces
¾ pound/340g zucchini (2 medium), cut into ½-inch/1cm cubes
¼ teaspoon salt
Freshly ground black pepper
¾ pound/340g deli roast beef, in ½-inch-thick slices, cut into ½-inch cubes
2 tablespoons Worcestershire sauce
4 large eggs
¼ cup grated Parmesan cheese

In a large nonstick skillet, heat the oil over medium heat. Add the onion and garlic, cover, and cook, stirring once or twice, until softened and beginning to brown, about 4 minutes. Add the water, asparagus, zucchini, salt, and a few grinds of pepper. Cover and steam until the asparagus is mostly tender, about 5 minutes. Add the roast beef and Worcestershire sauce and toss to coat. Crack an egg onto each of the four quarters of the pan. Reduce the heat to medium-low, cover, and cook until the egg whites are cooked and the yolks are to your liking, 7 to 8 minutes for runny yolks. Serve sprinkled with Parmesan and a few grinds of pepper.

OPTIONAL EXTRA: If you like spice, add a tablespoon (or two if you dare) of minced pickled jalapeños when you add the roast beef.

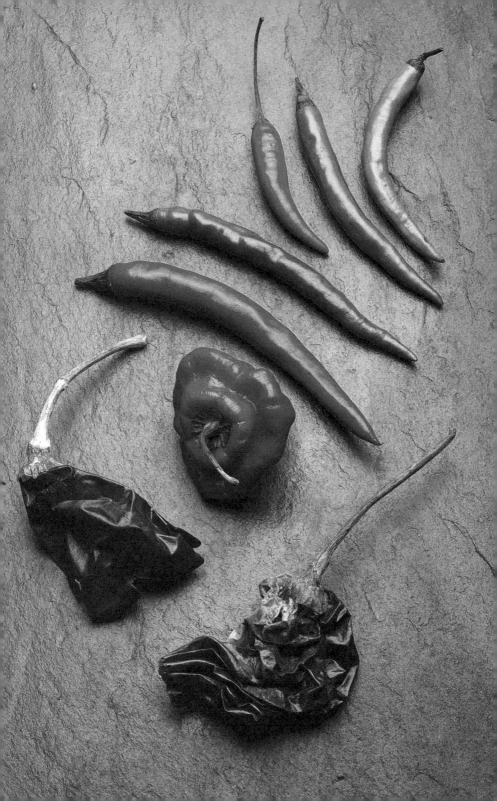

Lightning Quick

Really Fast Fast Food

There are days when life's a blur. These aren't the leisurely, luxury days when you can spend hours in the company of a recipe, sieving, dicing, and marinating, flour up to your elbows and your head in a cookbook. These are the real Fast Days. The evenings when you walk through the door, plunk down your bag, pick up a fork. What you want then is speed cooking. With just a little planning, you can eat well—and well within the FastDiet calorie quota—using ingredients hauled quickly from the cupboard or the fridge.

SHRIMP AND ASPARAGUS STIR-FRY

105 CALORIES PER PORTION

Serves 2

Once you've assembled your ingredients, the whole cooking process should be done in 6 minutes—which is not much longer than it would take to microwave a frozen dinner. And look at the calorie count. Minuscule.

1 teaspoon vegetable oil
1 medium onion, sliced
2 garlic cloves, crushed
1 teaspoon ground ginger
1 red bird's eye chile, seeded and finely chopped
4 scallions, finely sliced on the diagonal
1 lemongrass stalk, smashed
2 kaffir lime leaves
3 tablespoons Thai fish sauce
2 tablespoons boiling water
½ teaspoon sugar
12 raw jumbo shrimp
10 ounces/285g asparagus, halved lengthwise and cut into 1¼-inch/3cm pieces
Cilantro leaves, Thai basil leaves, lime wedges, for serving

Heat the oil in a wok, and stir-fry the onion, garlic, ginger, and chile until softened. Add the scallions, cook for another minute, add the lemongrass, lime leaves, fish sauce, water, and sugar. Stir, then add the shrimp and asparagus. Cook on high heat for 3 minutes, or until the shrimp is pink and the asparagus is al dente. Remove the lemongrass. Serve with fresh cilantro leaves, Thai basil, and a wedge of lime.

OPTIONAL EXTRAS: Add 3½ ounces/100g of halved baby corn (+25 calories) and sugar snaps (+35 calories) along with the asparagus for bulk and vibrant color.

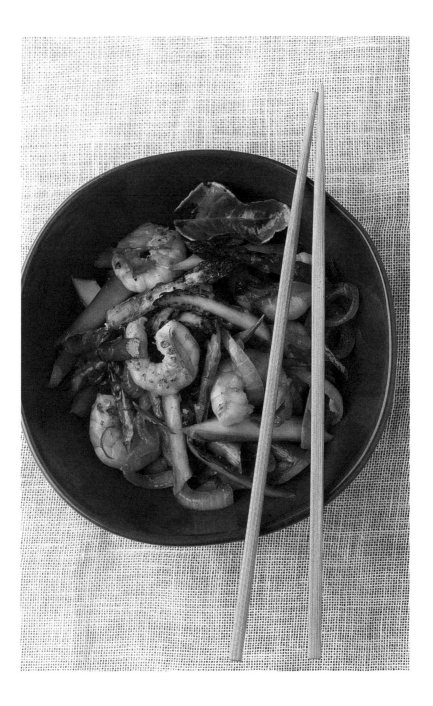

FAST DAY CHICKEN
SIX SPEEDY WAYS . . .

. . . with gremolata and dark leaves

140 CALORIES PER PORTION

Serves 4

Gremolata is a vivid green Italian sauce made from finely chopped garlic, lemon zest, and masses of parsley, traditionally served with osso buco, but a great way to dress up any plain grilled or seared meat or fish.

For the gremolata
Generous handful of fresh
   flat-leaf parsley, finely
   chopped
1 tablespoon extra-virgin olive oil
Zest of 1 lemon
1 tablespoon lemon juice
1 teaspoon finely chopped fresh
   oregano
1 teaspoon finely chopped fresh
   thyme leaves

2 garlic cloves, very finely
   chopped
Salt and freshly ground black
   pepper

4 skinless, boneless chicken thighs
   (about 7¾ ounces/220g each)
2 teaspoons olive oil
Salt and pepper
Dark salad leaves or blanched
   green beans, for serving

In a small bowl, combine the parsley, extra-virgin olive oil, lemon zest and juice, oregano, thyme, garlic, salt, and pepper. Stir well and set aside. Score the meat several times, drizzle with the olive oil and season well with salt and pepper, then place on a hot grill pan. Cook on medium heat until golden and sticky, then turn and cook until the meat is cooked through, about 5 minutes on each side. Serve drizzled with 1 tablespoon gremolata and a side of dark salad leaves such as watercress, arugula, mâche, baby spinach, or blanched green beans.

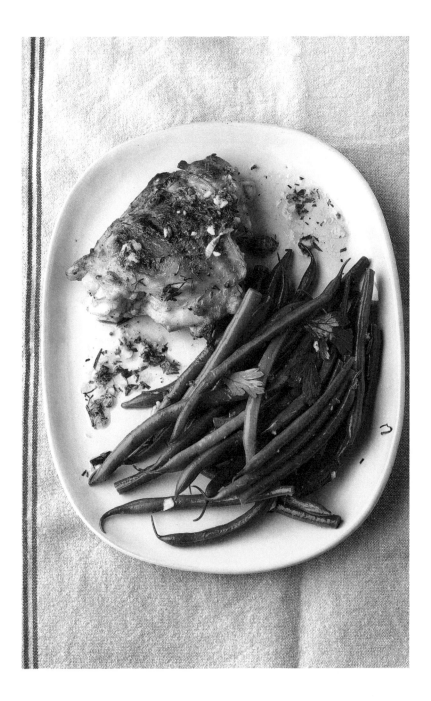

... Tex-Mex chicken

263 CALORIES PER PORTION

Serves 4

The most vital element for successful Fast Day cooking is accessing as much flavor as you can, for the fewest possible calories. Here, a rub of ancho chile powder, spices, herbs—plus a little sweet honey and a sharp, astringent kick of lime—raise this chicken staple out of the ordinary and into the sublime.

1 teaspoon ground coriander
¾ teaspoon ground cumin
½ teaspoon dried oregano
½ teaspoon sugar
¾ teaspoon ancho chile powder
¾ teaspoon coarse salt

4 skin-on, bone-in chicken breast halves (about 10 ounces/285g each)
2 tablespoons lime juice
2 teaspoons honey
1 tablespoon olive oil

Preheat the oven to 425°F. In a small bowl, combine the coriander, cumin, oregano, sugar, and ½ teaspoon each of the chile powder and salt. With your fingers, carefully lift the chicken skin without removing it and rub the spice mixture under the skin and all over the chicken. Place a rimmed baking sheet in the oven to heat for 5 minutes. Place the chicken skin side down in the pan and bake until the skin begins to brown, about 15 minutes. Turn the chicken over and bake until the chicken is just cooked through and registers 160°F on an instant read thermometer, 8 to 10 minutes longer. (The temperature will rise 5°F after the chicken comes out of the oven.) Meanwhile, in a small bowl, stir together the lime juice, honey, oil, and the remaining ¼ teaspoon each chile powder and salt. To serve, remove the skin and serve the chicken with the sauce.

● You can make a larger batch of the spice rub and store it on your spice shelf where it'll keep for 3 months. The rub is good on chicken, pork, beef, and shrimp.

● Cooking the chicken with the skin on keeps it moist, and since you remove it once the chicken has cooked, it doesn't add any calories.

. . . with peppers and capers

179 CALORIES PER PORTION

Serves 4

4 skinless, boneless chicken thighs (about 7¾ ounces/220g each), trimmed of excess fat, scored
1 teaspoon olive oil
Salt and freshly ground black pepper
2 red bell peppers, seeded and finely sliced
2 garlic cloves, sliced
1 sprig fresh rosemary
⅔ cup/150ml water
1 chicken bouillon cube
2 tablespoons capers, rinsed
7 ounces/200g baby spinach
Zest of 1 lemon, for serving

Drizzle the chicken with oil and season well, then place in a hot grill pan. Cook on medium heat until just golden, then turn and continue to brown for 3 to 4 minutes. Remove the chicken from the pan and set aside. Add the bell peppers, garlic, and rosemary to the pan and sauté for 3 to 4 minutes. Return the chicken to the pan, add the water and bouillon cube, and stir well to combine. Simmer for 20 minutes, or until the sauce is reduced a bit and the chicken is cooked through. Add the capers and spinach, and stir on the heat for another 2 minutes. Serve with a sprinkle of lemon zest.

... with Dijon marinade

210 CALORIES PER PORTION

Serves 2

One of my favorite answers to the perennial "what's for supper?" question—this is fast, tasty, and pleasingly low in fat.

10½ ounces/300g chicken tenders	1 tablespoon Dijon mustard
Salt and freshly ground black pepper	2 tablespoons low-fat plain yogurt
	2 teaspoons herbes de Provence
	Squeeze of lemon

Combine all the ingredients in a bowl and set aside. Grill the chicken pieces for 3 to 4 minutes on each side, or until they are cooked through and nicely striped. Serve with a squeeze of lemon and a simple green salad.

FAST DAY TIP: Marinate the chicken in a plastic bag in the morning or the previous night and refrigerate to infuse it with maximum flavor.

... with masala and raita

221 CALORIES PER PORTION

Serves 4

4 skinless chicken thighs (about
7¾ ounces/220g each), scored
1 cup/200g low-fat plain yogurt
2 tablespoons masala paste
2 garlic cloves, crushed
Salt and freshly ground black
pepper
Handful of fresh cilantro,
chopped
Zest and juice of 1 lime

For the raita
1 cup/200g low-fat plain yogurt
1 medium cucumber, peeled,
halved, seeded, and sliced
Fresh mint leaves
Squeeze of lemon
Salt and freshly ground black
pepper

Preheat the oven to 400°F. Combine the chicken with the yogurt, masala paste, garlic, salt, pepper, half the cilantro, the lime juice and zest in a bowl. Set aside in the fridge to marinate for 30 minutes, or more if you have time. Place the chicken in a small roasting pan and bake for 20 minutes, or until it is cooked through. Combine the raita ingredients and serve alongside the chicken, topped with more lime zest and a scatter of cilantro leaves.

FAST DAY TIP: You may want to cook the chicken with its skin on to retain the juice and flavor, but don't eat the skin. I prefer to remove most of the skin before marinating to get the flavor well absorbed into the meat.

FAST DAY TIP: The masala yogurt marinade also works well with a whole chicken; score the meat and cover with the marinade. Massage into the meat and marinate overnight. Cook in a preheated oven at 400°F until the juices run clear (1 to 1½ hours).

...Chinese spice

273 CALORIES PER PORTION

Serves 2

10½ ounces/300g chicken
   tenders
1 tablespoon soy sauce
1 tablespoon mirin
1 garlic clove, crushed
½ teaspoon Chinese five-spice
   powder

2 teaspoons honey
1 teaspoon sesame oil
2 star anise
Freshly ground black pepper
1 red chile, finely sliced (seeded
   to taste), for serving

Combine the ingredients in a bowl and set aside in the fridge (you can do this the night before if you get the chance—a longer marinating time will allow the flavors to develop more fully, but if you're strapped for time, it's fine to cook immediately). Grill the chicken pieces for 3 to 4 minutes on each side, or until they are cooked through and nicely striped. Season with plenty of pepper and serve with a scatter of red chile.

● Goes well with steamed bok choy (+12 calories per 3½ ounces/100g).

NO-FUSS FISH WITH CHILI DRESSING

175 CALORIES PER PORTION

Serves 2

For the dressing
1 red chile, seeded and very
    finely chopped
Pinch of sugar
2 tablespoons Thai fish sauce
2 tablespoons lemon juice
2 tablespoons chopped fresh
    flat-leaf parsley

Snipped fresh chives
2 fresh cod fillets (about
    7 ounces/200g each)
Cooking spray
Salt and freshly ground black
    pepper

Mix the dressing ingredients in a bowl. Preheat the oven to 400°F. Lightly coat an ovenproof casserole with cooking spray. Season the fillets with salt and pepper and steam or bake until cooked through and opaque, 12 to15 minutes. Spoon the dressing over the fish and serve with a simple green salad or plenty of steamed broccoli.

CHEAT'S TIP: Place the fish fillet in a microwaveable bowl, add slices of lemon, and cover with plastic wrap. Punch a hole in the plastic wrap and cook on full power until opaque, about 3 minutes.

● Goes well with Asian Sesame Salad, page 121 (+133 calories per portion).

PORK MILANESE WITH ARUGULA

299 CALORIES PER PORTION

Serves 4

Too good to be true on a Fast Day? Not if you're careful to remove the fat from your meat, and dress it in panko bread crumbs—these are larger and crunchier than regular store-bought bread crumbs, which makes for a particularly crisp coating without absorbing too much cooking fat (once you've opened the bag or box, you can store it in the freezer for several months). All you need is the peppery punch of arugula to make this the perfect, well-balanced midweek supper.

4 boneless pork loin chops (4 ounces/110g each)
½ teaspoon salt
¼ teaspoon freshly ground black pepper
1 tablespoon all-purpose flour
1 large egg white beaten with 1 tablespoon water
½ cup panko bread crumbs
3 tablespoons grated Parmesan cheese
Cooking spray
2 tablespoons fresh lemon juice
1 tablespoon extra-virgin olive oil
½ teaspoon Dijon mustard
4 cups arugula

Season the pork loin with the salt and pepper. Sprinkle the flour over the pork loin, patting it in. Dip the pork loin in the egg mixture, letting the excess drip off. In a shallow bowl, combine the panko bread crumbs and Parmesan. Dip the pork in the panko bread crumb mixture patting to adhere. Generously coat a large nonstick skillet with cooking spray and heat over medium heat. Add the pork loin and cook, turning the pork loin midway, until golden brown and cooked through, about 5 minutes total. Transfer to four serving plates. In a medium bowl, whisk together the lemon juice, oil, and mustard. Add the arugula and toss to combine. Top the pork loin with the arugula and serve.

• If you like, you can bread the pork loin several hours before cooking it and let it sit in the fridge. This will also help set the coating.

• The Parmesan gives just a little bit of flavor that is hard to identify but a nice flavoring agent for the panko bread crumbs. If you like, you can add some dried parsley or basil to the panko bread crumb mix.

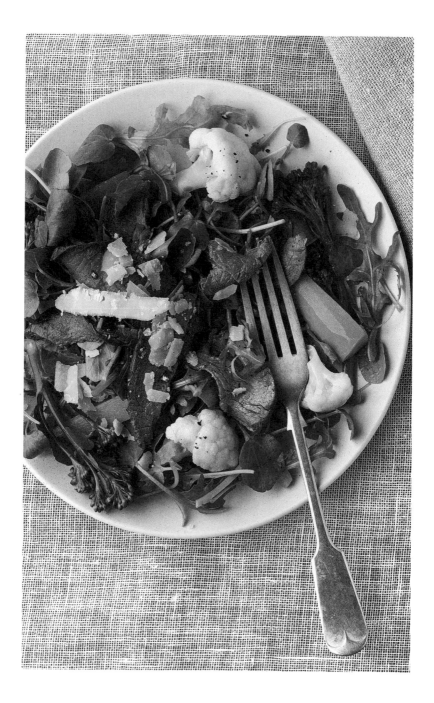

FIVE-MINUTE ROAST BEEF SALAD

248 CALORIES PER PORTION

Serves 2

This is grab-bag cooking. And none the worse for it.

8 ounces/240g frozen carrots, cauliflower, and broccoli florets

2 tablespoons Fast Day Dressing (page 143)

Generous handful of watercress and arugula leaves

3½ ounces/100g cooked roast beef slices—leftovers or store-bought, the thinner and rarer the better

2 tablespoons shaved Parmesan cheese

Salt and cracked black pepper

Microwave the vegetables in their bag on full power for 3 to 4 minutes. Remove from the bag and drizzle the dressing over the warm vegetables. Add the watercress and arugula, and top with strips of rare roast beef and shavings of fresh Parmesan. Season well with salt and pepper and serve.

CHICKPEA CURRY IN A HURRY

249 CALORIES PER PORTION

Serves 2

Five minutes. Two forks. Done.

Cooking spray
1 medium onion, diced
2 garlic cloves, crushed
3 teaspoons curry powder
¼ teaspoon red pepper flakes
Scant 1 cup/200ml boiling water
1 vegetable bouillon cube

2 tablespoons tomato paste
1 (14-ounce/400g) can chickpeas,
  rinsed and drained
Salt and freshly ground black
  pepper
1 tablespoon low-fat plain
  yogurt, for serving

Heat a pan and spray with oil. Add the onion and garlic and sauté until softened. Add the curry powder and red pepper flakes and cook for another 2 minutes. Add the boiling water, bouillon cube, tomato paste, and chickpeas. Simmer until the chickpeas are heated through and the sauce has thickened. Season and serve with a swirl of yogurt, and perhaps a salad of thinly sliced cucumber.

OPTIONAL EXTRAS: Add a handful of spinach leaves or 10 cherry tomatoes (+35 calories) for the last 2 minutes of cooking.

FAST DAY TIP: To make a curry with more complexity, add a cinnamon stick, 3 curry leaves, a clove, 1 teaspoon black mustard seeds, a halved chile, and a couple of cardamom pods to the pan with the sautéing onion; add 2 tablespoons of ground almonds (+70 calories) for a thicker curry sauce.

FISH TACOS

290 CALORIES PER PORTION

Serves 4

A great way to combine a trio of FastDiet favorites: lean protein, raw veggies—be generous—and tons of flavor. Go for whole-grain tortillas for a slower burn carb, and choose white fish over salmon, which is higher in calories.

½ cup/100g fat-free plain yogurt
1 tablespoon olive oil
  mayonnaise
1 pound/450g white fish fillets,
  such as cod, grouper, or
  snapper
1 tablespoon olive oil
1 tablespoon lime juice
½ teaspoon ground coriander

½ teaspoon salt
8 taco-size whole-grain flour
  tortillas
2 cups shredded cabbage
1 small red onion, halved and
  thinly sliced
1 medium plum tomato, diced
1 jalapeño pepper, thinly sliced

In a small bowl, stir together the yogurt and mayonnaise and refrigerate. Position a rack 4 inches from the heat source and preheat the broiler. Line a baking sheet with foil. In a bowl, toss the fish with the oil, lime juice, coriander, and salt. Place the fish on the baking sheet and broil until opaque throughout, about 5 minutes. Wrap the tortillas in foil and place in the oven while the broiler is on for 3 to 4 minutes to heat them up, or heat them in the microwave, wrapped in paper towels. Cut the fish into 16 strips. In a small bowl, toss together the cabbage, onion, tomato, and jalapeño. Fill each tortilla with the cabbage mixture. Top with the fish and the yogurt sauce.

● Mayonnaise made with olive oil is significantly lower in calories than regular full-fat mayo.

QUICK ROAST PORK LOIN WITH BROCCOLI, CAULIFLOWER, AND CHEESE SAUCE

386 CALORIES PER PORTION

Serves 4

I like the ease and relative fatlessness of a good pork tenderloin. Have it with cheesy veggies for a great supper on a cold day—or try it with any of the chicken accompaniments from pages 38–44.

1 pork tenderloin fillet (about 1 pound/450g)	5 ounces/150g cauliflower florets
1 teaspoon olive oil	5 ounces/150g broccoli florets
Salt and freshly ground black pepper	6 ounces/175g store-bought cheese sauce
2 teaspoons fennel seeds, crushed	1¾ ounces/50g sharp cheddar, grated

Preheat the oven to 400°F. Rub the pork loin with the oil, then season with salt and pepper, and roll in the fennel seeds. Place in a small roasting pan and bake for 20 to 25 minutes, depending on the thickness of the fillet, until cooked through. Cover with foil during cooking time if the meat is browning too much. Let rest. Meanwhile, boil, steam, or microwave the cauliflower and broccoli. Drain well and place in a small ovenproof dish. Heat the cheese sauce and pour over the drained vegetables—ensure that they are as dry as possible to prevent weeping. Top with the cheddar and place in a hot oven for 5 minutes to melt the cheese. Cut the pork into medallions, pour the pan juices on top, and serve with a gooey spoonful of cheesy veggies.

FAST DAY TIP: Use sharp rather than mild cheddar to maximize flavor and keep calories in check. Or use feta for its strong flavor and relatively low calorie count.

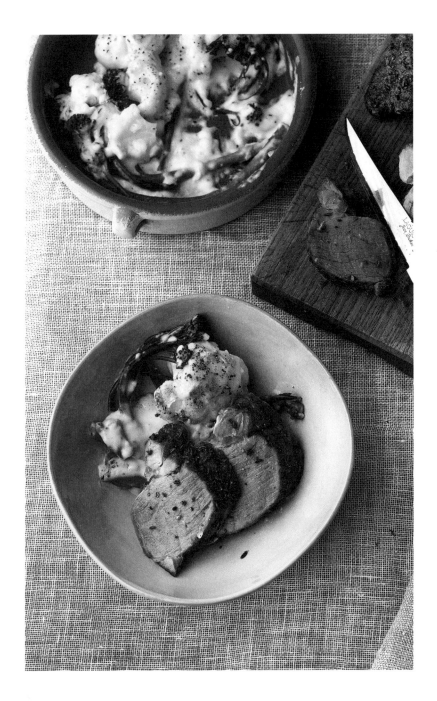

PEPPERED PORK WITH SUMMER SLAW

467 CALORIES PER PORTION

Serves 2

2 boneless pork chops (about
  5½ ounces/155g each)
1 teaspoon olive oil
Cracked black pepper
Sea salt

For the slaw
1 medium green apple, unpeeled
  and grated
¼ medium white cabbage,
  shredded
2 tablespoons chopped fresh
  chives
⅓ cup/75g low-fat crème fraîche
1 teaspoon honey
Juice of 1 lemon

Preheat the oven to 400°F. Rub the pork with the oil, season with the pepper and salt, and sear on all sides in a grill pan. Cover with foil. Turn off the oven and transfer the pan to the cooling oven for 8 to 10 minutes, or until the pork is cooked through. Remove from the oven and rest for 5 minutes. Combine the slaw ingredients, mix well, and serve alongside the pork.

OPTIONAL EXTRAS: Add 1 tablespoon golden raisins (+48 calories) and 1 tablespoon walnuts (+50 calories) to the slaw for extra sweetness and crunch.

. . . OR WITH WARM WINTER SLAW

493 CALORIES PER PORTION

Serves 2

2 boneless pork chops (about
    5½ ounces/155g each)
1 teaspoon olive oil
¼ teaspoon red pepper flakes
2 teaspoons cracked black
    pepper
½ teaspoon sea salt

For the slaw
¼ medium white cabbage, finely
    shredded
¼ medium red cabbage, finely
    shredded
1 medium carrot, peeled and
    julienned

2 scallions, finely sliced
1 tablespoon raisins
Handful of fresh cilantro

For the dressing
1 tablespoon sherry vinegar
1 tablespoon olive oil
1½ teaspoons walnut oil
1 teaspoon honey
¼ teaspoon red pepper flakes
1 garlic clove, crushed
Salt and freshly ground black
    pepper

Preheat the oven to 400°F. Rub the pork with the olive oil. Combine the red pepper flakes, black pepper, and salt in a small bowl and sprinkle over the meat. Heat an ovenproof grill pan and sear the pork for 2 minutes on each side. Cover with foil. Turn off the oven and transfer the grill pan to the cooling oven for 8 to 10 minutes, or until cooked through. Remove from the oven and rest for 5 minutes. Meanwhile, put the slaw ingredients in a bowl. Combine the dressing ingredients in a small saucepan and gently warm through. Pour on the salad ingredients and toss well. Check the seasoning. Serve in a plentiful mound alongside the pork.

FAST DAY OMELETS

... plain

150 to 190 CALORIES, DEPENDING ON SIZE OF EGGS

Serves 1

There are few square meals that can beat an omelet on a Fast Day. Swift. Tasty. Filling. And all done in one lone pan.

    2 medium eggs
    Salt and freshly ground black pepper
    Cooking spray

Beat the eggs with a fork until bubbly. Add salt and plenty of pepper, lightly coat a small frying pan with cooking spray, and cook gently until the omelet is set to your liking.

... or try an omelet with:

- 1 teaspoon curry spices added to the egg mix **+0 calories**

- 1 tablespoon finely chopped pimientos **+10 calories**

- 1¾ ounces/50g cooked shrimp and 1 tablespoon chopped cilantro **+45 calories**

- 1 tablespoon ricotta and a handful of spinach leaves **+46 calories**

- 3½ ounces/100g lightly steamed or microwaved mushrooms (drained) and a scatter of freshly chopped parsley **+55 calories**

- 1 tablespoon cooked crabmeat and 1 tablespoon shaved Parmesan cheese **+55 calories**

- 1 chopped scallion and ¼ teaspoon red pepper flakes, lightly sautéed, topped with 2 teaspoons/10g crumbled goat cheese and a handful of chopped fresh parsley **+66 calories**

- steamed asparagus topped with 2 torn slices of prosciutto **+75 calories**

- 1¾ ounces/50g smoked trout, 1 finely sliced scallion, 1 teaspoon chopped fresh dill, and 1 tablespoon low-fat cream cheese **+85 calories**

- 1¾ ounces/50g low-fat mozzarella, 4 sliced canned artichoke hearts, and a chopped ripe tomato **+85 calories**

- 1¾ ounces/50g feta cheese, 3 chopped black olives, and a scatter of fresh sage **+120 calories**

- 1¾ ounces/50g torn smoked salmon and chopped chives topped with a swirl of low-fat crème fraîche just before serving, perhaps with 1 teaspoon rinsed capers **+160 calories**

- 1¾ ounces/50g crumbled chèvre and 1 tablespoon Homemade Oven-Dried Tomatoes (page 145) **+182 calories**

- 1¾ ounces/50g grated sharp cheddar and 1¾ ounces/50g frozen baby peas **+275 calories**

STRAIGHT TO THE PLATE . . .

Not recipes so much as great flavor combinations, these can be grabbed from your fridge and kitchen cupboards on days when you don't want to think too hard about food (or indeed precise calorie counts. . . . All the below are Fast Day friendly suggestions). Just add the simple Fast Day Dressing from page 143 where desired or required.

- smoked fish fillet, arugula, plum tomatoes

- canned tuna, cannellini beans, red onion

- roast beef, grilled halloumi, arugula

- avocado, cooked shrimp, plain yogurt

- mozzarella, avocado, ripe tomato

- sliced ham or prosciutto, melon, strawberries

- blanched green beans, cooked jumbo shrimp, feta

- hummus, raw veggies, jalapeños

- white cabbage, red onion, hard-boiled egg

- smoked chicken, romaine lettuce, cashews

- sardines, cherry tomatoes, steamed broccoli florets

- beef carpaccio, toasted pine nuts, arugula, Parmesan

- lean roast beef, horseradish crème fraîche, Boston lettuce

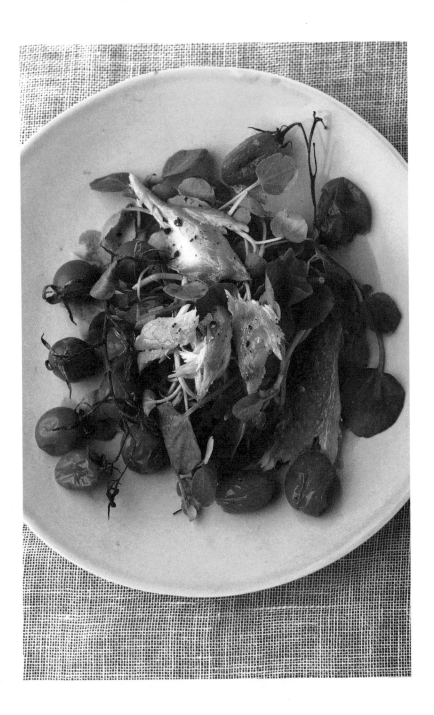

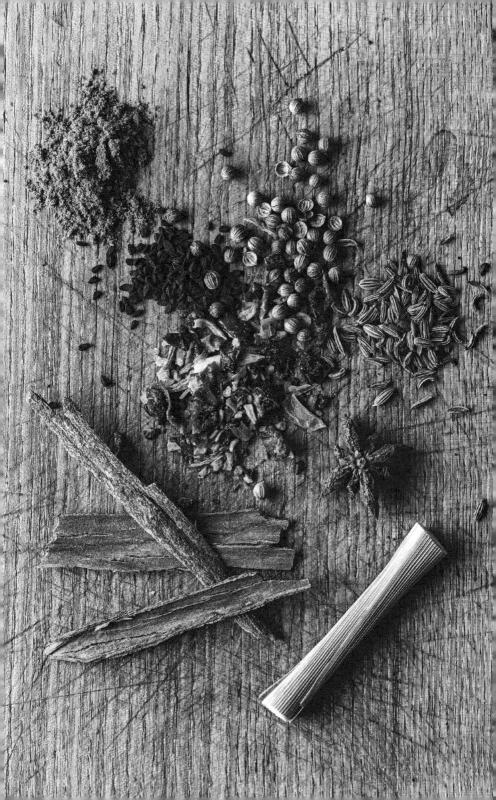

Warming and Wonderful

Comfort Food for Hungry Days

If you've been on the FastDiet for some time, you may well have had your fill of salad leaves. So, what about the days when you're in need of something warm, something substantial, the culinary equivalent of a cuddle? That's where these stews, curries, and casseroles come in. You'll know them all, but here, well-loved recipes have been relieved of superfluous calories to make them ideal for a Fast Day. Many are freezer friendly, so make them in bulk and store them.

CHICKEN AND CABBAGE CHOP SUEY

264 CALORIES PER PORTION

Serves 4

This super-simple Chinese American dish often gets overlooked, but its straightforward flavors are surprisingly satisfying. This chop suey delivers a quick and tasty midweek supper, made FastDiet friendly by replacing the noodles with shredded cabbage. You get a sweetness and tenderness by cooking it this way. Noodles? Who needs noodles?

1 tablespoon extra-virgin olive oil

1¼ pounds/565g boneless, skinless chicken breasts, thinly sliced

3 cups finely shredded red cabbage

4 large celery stalks, thinly sliced on an angle

1 cup finely sliced red onion

10 ounces/285g white mushrooms, thinly sliced

6 tablespoon water

½ teaspoon salt

2 tablespoons all-purpose flour

¼ teaspoon freshly ground black pepper

2 tablespoons reduced-sodium soy sauce, plus more for serving

In a nonstick Dutch oven, heat the oil over high heat. Add the chicken and cook until just beginning to turn opaque on the surface, 1 to 2 minutes. Reduce the heat to medium-high and add the cabbage, celery, onion, mushrooms, and 3 tablespoons of the water. Sprinkle with the salt. Stir to combine, cover, and cook, stirring frequently, until the cabbage has softened, 6 to 8 minutes. In a small bowl, combine the flour and pepper. Stir in the soy sauce and the remaining 3 tablespoons water until the mixture is smooth. Push the cabbage to one side of the Dutch oven and add the soy sauce mixture. Stir to combine with the vegetables and cook, uncovered and stirring often, until the sauce thickens and coats the ingredients, about 2 minutes. Serve hot with soy sauce on the side.

OPTIONAL EXTRAS: Although the classic dish is traditionally tame in flavor, you could always spike it with a little chili-garlic sauce, such as Sriracha. Add a small squeeze to the soy sauce mixture that gets added at the end. And you could garnish the dish with chopped cilantro.

COD ARRABBIATA

220 CALORIES PER PORTION

Serves 4

The Italian word *arrabbiata* means "angry"—and in the case of this sauce, it refers to the spiciness that comes from hot peppers. Canned fire-roasted tomatoes come in several varieties and I've used one with green chiles—spicy, but not killer hot. If you prefer, you can use two cans of regular diced tomatoes and add your own heat. But do go as angry as you dare . . .

1 tablespoon olive oil
1 medium yellow bell pepper,
   seeded and cut into 1-inch
   squares
½ cup finely chopped onion
3 garlic cloves, thinly sliced
2 (14-ounce/400g) cans diced

fire-roasted tomatoes
  with chiles
½ teaspoon salt
1½ pounds/700g thick cod fillets,
  cut into 4 pieces
Cracked black pepper

In a large skillet, heat the oil over medium heat. Add the bell pepper, onion, and garlic and cook, stirring frequently, until the bell pepper and onion are tender, about 7 minutes. Add the tomatoes and salt and bring to a boil. Reduce to a simmer and cook, stirring occasionally, until the sauce is the consistency of a thick tomato sauce, about 10 minutes. Place the fish on top, cover, and cook until the fish is just cooked through, 7 to 10 minutes. Sprinkle the black pepper over the top and serve.

THREE TAGINES . . .

There's plenty of warmth and tenderness here. Unleash the fragrant aromas with a flourish of the lid as you serve.

. . . chicken tagine with preserved lemons and saffron

162 CALORIES PER PORTION

Serves 4

Cooking spray

4 skinless, bone-in chicken thighs (about 7¾ ounces/220g each)

2 medium onions, finely chopped

1 medium celery stalk, finely chopped

3 garlic cloves, crushed

4 medium ripe tomatoes, seeded and sliced

1½ cups/350ml chicken stock

½ teaspoon saffron threads

½ teaspoon ground turmeric

½ teaspoon ground cumin

½ teaspoon paprika

1 teaspoon ground coriander

1 teaspoon honey

1¼-inch/3cm piece fresh ginger, peeled and grated

1 cinnamon stick

2 small preserved lemons, finely chopped

1 teaspoon harissa paste

Salt and freshly ground black pepper

Squeeze of lemon, handful of chopped fresh cilantro leaves and pomegranate seeds, for serving

Heat a little oil in a tagine or large ovenproof casserole, add the chicken pieces and brown all over. Add the onions, celery, and garlic and sweat on low heat for 10 minutes, stirring occasionally. Add the tomatoes, stock, saffron, turmeric, cumin, paprika, coriander, honey, ginger, cinnamon stick, preserved lemons, and harissa paste. Stir, cover, and simmer for 1½ hours. Season well. Just before serving, shred the chicken off the bone and return to the pot. Serve garnished with a squeeze of lemon, plenty of cilantro, and pomegranate seeds.

... vegetable tagine with herbed couscous

311 CALORIES PER PORTION

Serves 4

For the tagine
1 tablespoon olive oil
2 medium onions, thinly sliced
2 teaspoons ground cumin
2 teaspoons ground coriander
1 teaspoon ground ginger
2 garlic cloves, crushed
2 tablespoons harissa paste
2 medium carrots, peeled and
   cut into chunks
2 medium parsnips, about 1
   pound/450g, peeled and cut
   into chunks
1 small butternut squash (about
   1 pound/450g), peeled, seeded,
   and cut into chunks
Salt and freshly ground black
   pepper

2 cups/500ml vegetable stock or
   boiling water and a vegetable
   bouillon cube
2½ ounces/75g dried apricots,
   chopped
1 tablespoon lemon juice
1 (14-ounce/400g) can chickpeas,
   rinsed and drained

For the couscous
10½ ounces/300g couscous
1 tablespoon pine nuts, toasted
Small bunch of fresh flat-leaf
   parsley, chopped
Small bunch of fresh cilantro,
   chopped, and lemon zest, for
   serving

Heat the oil in a tagine or large ovenproof casserole, add the onions and cook for 5 minutes, until softened. Add the spices and garlic and cook for another minute. Add the harissa paste and vegetables, season, and stir well. Pour in the stock, add the apricots and lemon juice, and simmer for 30 minutes. Add the chickpeas and continue cooking for 10 minutes more. Prepare the couscous as per package directions, let stand for 10 minutes, fluff up with a fork, and add the pine nuts and herbs. Serve the tagine and couscous in a deep bowl, scattered with cilantro and lemon zest.

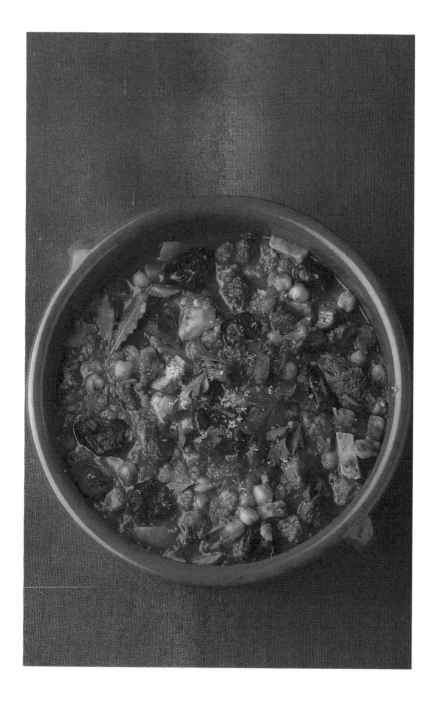

. . . Moroccan spiced lamb

349 CALORIES PER PORTION

Serves 4

1¼ pounds/565g leg of lamb, deboned, trimmed of fat, and cut into 1¼-inch/3cm cubes

Salt and freshly ground black pepper

Cooking spray

2 medium onions, peeled and sliced

2 garlic cloves, crushed

2 teaspoons ground cumin

2 teaspoons ground coriander

½ teaspoon ground cinnamon

1 teaspoon chili powder

1 (14-ounce/400g) can diced tomatoes

1¾ cups/400ml boiling water

1 beef bouillon cube

2 tablespoons honey

1 (14-ounce/400g) can chickpeas, rinsed and drained

1 bay leaf

1 medium sweet potato (about 7 ounces/200g), peeled and cut into 1¼-inch/3cm chunks

1¾ ounces/50g pitted prunes, halved

Generous handful of fresh flat-leaf parsley and lemon zest, for serving

Preheat the oven to 350°F. Season the lamb chunks with salt and pepper. Heat a large ovenproof casserole coated with a little cooking spray and sauté the lamb, onions, and garlic for 2 to 3 minutes, or until lightly browned. Add the spices, stir, and cook for another 2 minutes. Add the tomatoes, boiling water, crumbled bouillon cube, honey, chickpeas, and bay leaf. Stir well and bring to a simmer on the stove. Cover with a tight-fitting lid and transfer to the oven. Cook for 1 hour, then add the sweet potato and prunes, return to the oven, and cook for another 45 minutes. Serve sprinkled with parsley and lemon zest.

● Goes well with saffron and shallot sauce: mix 1/4 cup low-fat plain yogurt with a finely chopped shallot and a few saffron strands. Season and serve on the side (+25 calories per tablespoon).

NEAPOLITAN CIANFOTTA

179 CALORIES PER PORTION

Serves 4

This is a loose, family-style recipe for a delicious summer vegetable stew; use what you have and what you like. *Cianfotta* means "tasty and colorful," so keep it light and bright, without too many starchy vegetables. If you like capers, add a teaspoon or two along with the stock for a salty kick.

2 tablespoons olive oil
1 medium onion, finely diced
1 medium celery stalk, finely chopped
1 medium carrot, peeled and finely diced
3 garlic cloves, crushed
1 medium fennel bulb, trimmed and cut into 8 wedges
Handful of fresh marjoram or oregano, coarsely chopped
1 bay leaf
1 small eggplant, cut into ¾-inch/2cm cubes

4 medium zucchini, sliced into ¾-inch/2cm rounds
Salt and freshly ground black pepper
1¾ cups/400ml hot vegetable stock
7 ounces/200g cherry tomatoes, halved
7 ounces/200g sugar snap peas
7 ounces/200g snow peas
3½ ounces/100g frozen baby peas
4 zucchini flowers (if available)
Pecorino cheese, for serving

Preheat the oven to 350°F. Heat the oil in a large ovenproof casserole and sauté the onion until softened. Add the celery, carrot, garlic, fennel, marjoram, and bay leaf, cover, and sweat for another 5 minutes. Then add the eggplant and zucchini, season, stir, cover, and transfer to the oven for 30 minutes, stirring occasionally to release any stickiness from the pan base. Remove from the oven, add the vegetable stock and bring to a simmer. Add the cherry tomatoes, sugar snaps, snow peas, and baby peas. Season to taste, bring back to a simmer for 3 to 4 minutes, or until the vegetables are just cooked. Serve in deep soup bowls, with a decorative shaving of pecorino (+25 calories per tablespoon).

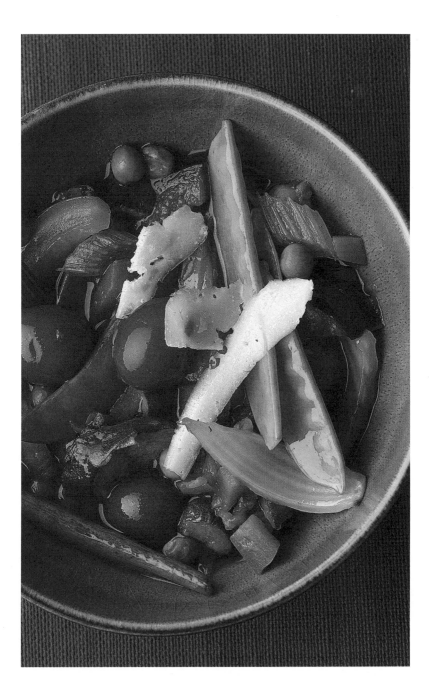

ONE-POT BEAN FEAST

207 CALORIES PER PORTION

Serves 4

Beans are a great source of low-fat, high-fiber protein. Play around with different types for a change of texture, taste, and color. You can buy a can of three-bean salad to get a good mix in a single can.

1 tablespoon olive oil
1 large red onion, chopped
2 garlic cloves, crushed
2 medium carrots, peeled and chopped
2 medium celery stalks, chopped
1 tablespoon fresh thyme leaves, or 1 teaspoon dried
2 (14-ounce/400g) cans mixed beans (cannellini, kidney, pinto, black beans), rinsed and drained

1 (14-ounce/400g) can diced tomatoes
1 tablespoon red wine vinegar
1 tablespoon honey
1 tablespoon Dijon mustard
Salt and freshly ground black pepper
1 sprig fresh rosemary
Generous handful of fresh parsley, chopped
1 cup/250ml water
Juice of 1 lime

Heat the oil in a large pan and sauté the onion and garlic until soft. Add the carrots, celery, and thyme and cook for another 5 minutes. Add the beans, tomatoes, vinegar, honey, mustard, salt, pepper, rosemary, half the parsley, and water. Stir, bring to a simmer, and cook, loosely covered, for 2 hours, stirring every half hour. Remove from the heat and add the lime juice and the remaining parsley. Serve with a lemon-dressed leaf salad and plenty of pepper.

FIRE AND SPICE VEGGIE CASSEROLE

247 CALORIES PER PORTION

Serves 4

1 teaspoon cumin seeds
1 teaspoon coriander seeds
1 teaspoon black mustard
  seeds
2 tablespoons olive oil
3 medium onions, sliced
3 medium carrots, peeled and
  coarsely chopped
2 medium leeks, trimmed and
  sliced
2 garlic cloves, crushed
1¼-inch/3cm piece fresh ginger,
  peeled and finely chopped

1 red chile, finely chopped
  (seeded to taste)
1 teaspoon chili powder
¼ teaspoon ground turmeric
7 ounces/200g split red lentils
1 pound/450g button
  mushrooms, halved
3¼ cups/750ml boiling water
1 vegetable bouillon cube
Salt and freshly ground black
  pepper
Handful of fresh cilantro,
  chopped

Crush the seeds in a mortar and pestle. Heat the oil in a large ovenproof casserole, add the onions, carrots, and leeks and sauté for 5 minutes. Add the garlic, ginger, red chile, chili powder, turmeric, and crushed spices and sauté for another 2 minutes. Stir in the lentils and mushrooms, add the boiling water, and the bouillon cube. Season, stir, cover, and simmer for 45 minutes to 1 hour. Stir in the cilantro before serving.

● Goes well with Tabbouleh, page 117 (+123 calories per portion).

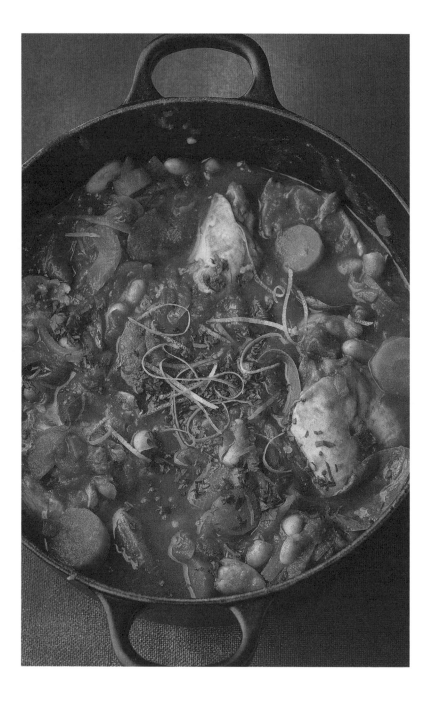

CHICKEN CASSOULET

318 CALORIES PER PORTION

Serves 4

Cassoulet is hearty, rustic, and full of beans. It usually contains plenty of fat—sausage, lardons, duck confit, pork skin, and the rest—but here, I've slimmed it down so that it fits snugly into a Fast Day. A little chorizo, though not French (*sacré bleu!*), will add depth. It's the slow cooking that lends the required unctuousness, so prep in advance and give it some time to develop.

1 tablespoon olive oil
2 medium onions, sliced
2 medium celery stalks, chopped
1¾ ounces/50g sausage, chopped
2 tablespoons tomato paste
8 garlic cloves, unpeeled and left whole
2 bay leaves
Scant ½ cup/100ml white wine
Scant ½ cup/100ml boiling water
Juice of ½ lemon
3 medium carrots, peeled and sliced into ½-inch/1cm rounds

1 (14-ounce/400g) can diced tomatoes
Salt and freshly ground black pepper
4 skinless, bone-in chicken thighs (about 7¾ ounces/220g each)
1 bouquet garni
1 (14-ounce/400g) can cannellini beans
Handful of fresh parsley, finely chopped, for serving

Preheat the oven to 350°F. Heat the oil in a large ovenproof pan, and cook the onions and celery over low heat for 2 to 3 minutes. When softened, add the sausage and sauté for another minute, or until it has browned. Add the tomato paste, garlic, and bay leaves, stir, and cook for another 5 minutes. Add the wine, water, and lemon juice, then simmer for 3 minutes to reduce a little. Add the carrots and tomatoes and season. Bring back to a simmer, then add the chicken, bouquet garni, and beans. Stir to coat well in the sauce and transfer to the oven for 1 to 1½ hours, until the chicken is cooked, tender, and falling off the bone. Just before serving, remove the bouquet garni, and mash some of the soft, sweet garlic cloves into the beans and sauce. Scatter with parsley and serve.

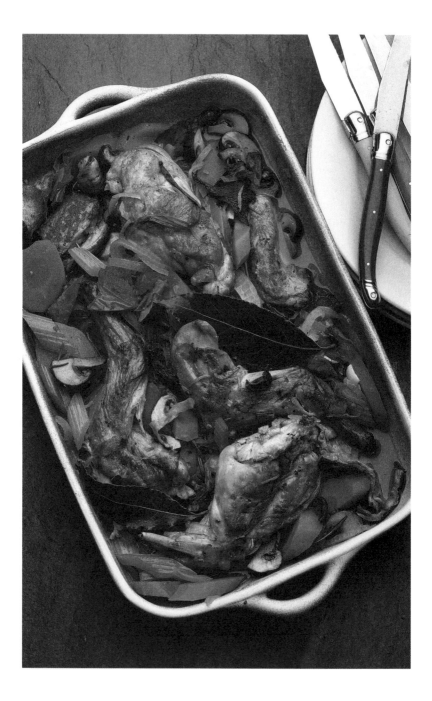

ITALIAN RABBIT STEW

328 CALORIES PER PORTION

Serves 4

Rabbit was once a regular on the UK's dinner tables; having fallen out of favor for decades, it's now firmly back on the menu. And there are very good reasons to try it: Rabbit can generally be locally sourced (ask your butcher), it's a comparatively sustainable source of meat, relatively low in fat and satisfyingly cheap.

2 tablespoons olive oil	2 bay leaves
1 rabbit (about 2 pounds/900g), cut into portions	Scant 1 cup/200ml white wine
1 medium onion, finely sliced	5 ounces/150g mushrooms, coarsely chopped
4 scallions, chopped	Scant 1 ounce/25g dried porcini mushrooms, rehydrated in boiling water for 15 minutes and drained
2 medium celery stalks, chopped	
2 medium carrots, peeled and chopped	
4 garlic cloves, crushed	3 medium ripe tomatoes, chopped
1 teaspoon capers	Juice and zest of 1 lemon
½ teaspoon fresh thyme leaves	Salt and cracked black pepper
2 sprigs fresh rosemary	
1 teaspoon dried oregano	

Preheat the oven to 350°F. Heat the oil in a large ovenproof casserole, season the rabbit, and sauté to brown on all sides. Add all the other ingredients except the lemon zest, stir to combine any stickiness from the pan base and bring to a simmer. Cover with a tight-fitting lid and transfer to the oven. Cook for 1 hour, or until the rabbit is tender and the sauce has become flavorful and rich. Serve garnished with the lemon zest and pepper.

● If rabbit is hard to come by, this dish can be made equally well with chicken.

● Goes well with Baked Fennel with Parmesan and Thyme, page 119 (+123 calories per portion), or Cannellini Bean Mash, page 122 (+183 calories per portion).

CHICKEN PROVENÇAL

348 CALORIES PER PORTION

Serves 4

Another French classic—just slim-line.

8 skinless, boneless chicken
thighs (7¾ ounces/220g each),
cut in half
Cooking spray
2 medium onions, sliced
2 garlic cloves, crushed
1 (14-ounce/400g) can diced
tomatoes
2 tablespoons tomato paste
⅔ cup/150ml chicken stock or
boiling water and a chicken
bouillon cube

2 teaspoons herbes de Provence
Scant ½ cup/100ml red wine
1 medium red bell pepper,
seeded and cut into chunks
1 medium yellow bell pepper,
seeded and cut into chunks
2 medium zucchini, cut into
¾-inch/2cm rounds
Salt and freshly ground black
pepper

Trim any excess fat off the chicken and season well. Coat a large nonstick frying pan with cooking spray and sauté the chicken over medium heat for 5 to 6 minutes, or until lightly browned. Add the onions, garlic, tomatoes, tomato paste, stock, herbes de Provence, and wine. Stir well. Bring to a simmer and cook for 10 minutes, stirring occasionally. Add the bell peppers and zucchini, bring back to a simmer, then cover and cook for 20 to 25 minutes, or until the chicken is cooked through. Season and serve.

● This sauce is delicious with jumbo shrimp, too; use 14 ounces/400g raw shrimp instead of the chicken and cook for 15 minutes in total.

● Goes well with Spring Cabbage with Mustard Seeds, page 111 (+27 calories per portion).

CHICKEN SAUSAGE JAMBALAYA

370 CALORIES PER PORTION

Serves 4

You get a lot of bang for your buck with this remodeled classic—tons of flavor, tons of color, and a veritable veggie carnival on your plate.

2 cups plus 2 tablespoons water
¾ cup brown basmati rice
4 garlic cloves, minced
½ teaspoon salt
Freshly ground black pepper
2 teaspoons extra-virgin olive oil
2 slices smoked Canadian bacon, minced
2 large green bell peppers, seeded and chopped

3 medium celery stalks with leaves, chopped
2 bunches scallions (including 2 inches of dark green), chopped, light and dark parts kept separate
1 pint/450g grape tomatoes, chopped
12 ounces/340g spicy chicken sausage, thinly sliced

Bring the 2 cups of the water, the rice, half the garlic, the salt, and a generous amount of black pepper to a boil in a small pot. Reduce to a simmer, partially cover, and cook for 20 minutes. Meanwhile, in a nonstick Dutch oven, heat the oil over medium-high heat. Add the Canadian bacon and cook until fragrant, about 1 minute. Add the bell peppers, celery, scallion whites, the remaining garlic, and the 2 tablespoons water. Reduce to a simmer, cover, and cook, stirring once or twice, until the vegetables are softened, about 8 minutes. Add the tomatoes and cook, uncovered, until the tomatoes collapse and get saucy, about 3 minutes. Add the rice mixture and any remaining cooking liquid and stir well. Let the mixture come to a simmer, then cover tightly and cook until the rice is tender, 8 to 10 minutes. Stir once or twice to be sure the jambalaya is not sticking. Stir in the sausage. Cover and cook until heated through, 3 to 5 minutes. Serve the jambalaya sprinkled with the reserved scallion greens.

● Use any kind of fully cooked spicy chicken sausage, though for a more authentic jambalaya try an andouille-style sausage. Chorizo-style chicken sausage would also be nice.

CHICKEN SALSA VERDE

293 CALORIES PER PORTION

Serves 4

As simple as it gets: lean chicken, punchy sauce. You can serve this on its own, or fill a plate with salad greens, top with the chicken, and spoon the sauce over it, making a delicious dressing for the greens.

1 pound/450g tomatillos, husks removed and tomatillos rinsed

¼ medium onion

1 jalapeño pepper, stemmed

2 garlic cloves

¼ cup packed chopped fresh cilantro leaves and tender stems

¾ teaspoon salt

2 teaspoons olive oil

4 skinless, boneless chicken breast halves (about 7 ounces/200g each)

In a medium saucepan, combine the tomatillos, onion, and jalapeño. Add water to cover and bring to a boil over medium heat. Reduce to a simmer and cook until the tomatillos are tender and pale green, about 5 minutes. Drain well and transfer to a blender along with the garlic, cilantro, and ¼ teaspoon of the salt. Blend until slightly chunky. In a large nonstick skillet, heat the oil over medium heat. Sprinkle the chicken with the remaining ½ teaspoon salt, add it to the pan, and cook for 2 minutes. Turn the chicken over, add the tomatillo mixture, and simmer uncovered, until the chicken is cooked through, about 7 minutes. Serve the chicken with the sauce spooned on top.

● Look for tomatillos in the produce section of the supermarket.

● Depending on the jalapeño, this sauce could end up more than a little spicy. If this is a concern, once the jalapeño has cooked, taste a small bit of it before pureeing the sauce. On the other hand, if you really like heat, try swapping in a serrano for the jalapeño.

BEEF AND BEER CASSEROLE

398 CALORIES PER PORTION

Serves 4

Cooking spray
2 medium onions, coarsely
  chopped
2 tablespoons all-purpose flour
Salt and freshly ground black
  pepper
2 teaspoons dried mixed herbs
2¼ pounds/1kg lean stewing
  beef, trimmed of fat and cut
  into 1 ¼-inch/3cm cubes

1 bay leaf
2 cups/500ml dark ale
1 cup/250ml beef stock or boiling
  water and bouillon cube
1 tablespoon tomato paste
3 medium carrots, peeled and
  sliced into ¾-inch/2cm rounds
1 pound/450g button
  mushrooms, halved if large

Preheat the oven to 350°F. Coat a pan with a little cooking spray and sauté the onions for 4 to 5 minutes. Combine the flour, salt, pepper, and mixed herbs. Dust the beef in the flour mixture, then place the beef in a large casserole dish with the onions, bay leaf, ale, stock, and tomato paste. Cover and cook in the oven for 2 to 2½ hours, adding the carrots and mushrooms for the last hour, then serve.

● Goes well with Spiced Red Cabbage with Apples, page 115 (+79 calories per portion), or any of the mash alternatives, pages 122–123.

BOSTON BEANS AND HAM

401 CALORIES PER PORTION

Serves 4

You'll get an unctuous, sticky plate of good food from this recipe. Go slow and savor.

1¾ pounds/850g smoked ham, bone-in
Cooking spray
1 medium onion, finely chopped
1 garlic clove, crushed
1 tablespoon tomato paste
2 tablespoons maple syrup
2 teaspoons English mustard powder
¼ teaspoon red pepper flakes
1 teaspoon paprika
½ teaspoon ground cinnamon
2 (14-ounce/400g) cans pinto beans, rinsed and drained
1¼ cups/300ml chicken or vegetable stock
Freshly ground black pepper

Preheat the oven to 350°F. Soak the ham in cold water for 15 minutes to release some of its saltiness. Dry well. Either leave the rind and string on, or remove it; you can also cut the ham in half to aid cooking (trimmed weight should be about 1½ pounds/700g). Spray an ovenproof casserole with oil and sauté the ham over medium heat until browned on all sides. Remove the ham from the pan and set aside on paper towels. Add the onion to the casserole and sauté for 2 minutes, stirring well to release the meat flavors from the pan base. Add the garlic, tomato paste, maple syrup, mustard powder, red pepper flakes, paprika, and cinnamon. Stir well and cook for another minute, then add the beans and stock and heat through. Add the ham, cover with a tight-fitting lid, and transfer to the oven for 45 to 50 minutes, removing the lid for the final 10 minutes to reduce the sauce. Season well with black pepper, check for saltiness, then remove the ham. Serve it sliced on top of the beans with some steamed, iron-rich greens to cut through the richness of the stew.

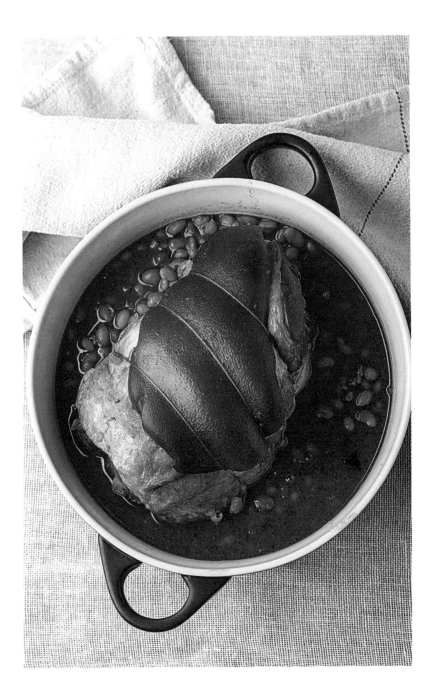

BEEF DAUBE WITH PEPPERED GREENS

429 CALORIES PER PORTION

Serves 4

The slow cooking here intensifies the flavor without requiring too much fat. I like the idea of dark vegetables with this—an earthy tangle of steamed kale, purple sprouting broccoli, or grilled radicchio would be perfect. The orange zest is an essential component—and do be generous with the pepper.

2¼ pounds/1kg lean braising beef, trimmed of fat and cut into 1¼-inch/3cm cubes
2 tablespoons all-purpose flour
Salt and freshly ground black pepper
1 large red onion, sliced
4 garlic cloves, crushed
1 (14-ounce/400g) can diced tomatoes
2 medium carrots, peeled and cut into ½-inch/1cm chunks
3 sprigs fresh thyme

1 bay leaf
Juice of 1 medium orange
1½ cups/350ml white wine
1¾ cups/400ml beef stock or boiling water and bouillon cube
4 anchovies, finely chopped
1¾ ounces/50g black olives
1 pound/450g curly kale or spring greens
Zest of ½ orange and cracked black pepper, for serving

Preheat the oven to 350°F. Toss the beef in well-seasoned flour and place in a large casserole along with all the other ingredients except the greens and the orange zest. Bring to a simmer, stir, cover with a tight-fitting lid, and then transfer to the oven. Cook until the beef is tender and the sauce thickened, 2 to 3 hours. Serve with steamed greens, a grating of orange zest, and a final flourish of cracked black pepper.

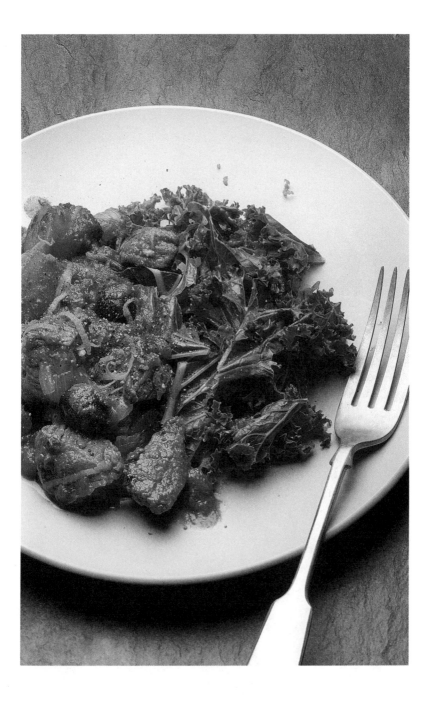

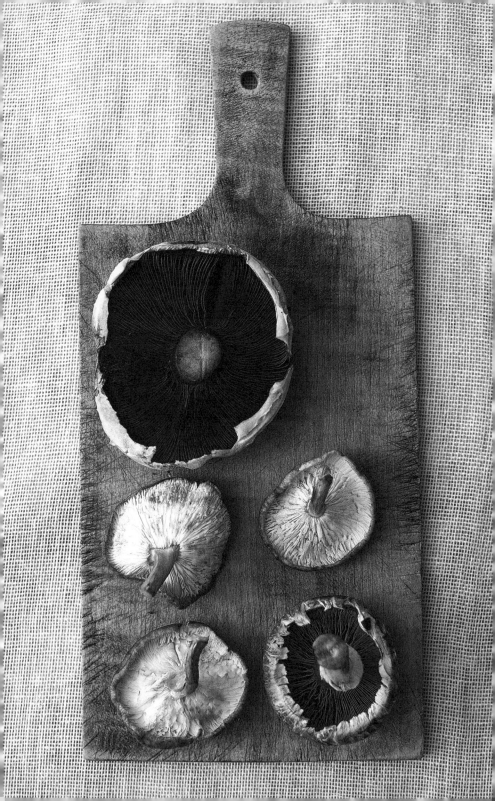

Fast-600

Filling Fast Day Meals for Men

As a historical rule, men don't tend to be wild about dieting. They don't like the hassle—all that counting and measuring, the eating from dolly plates, and saying no to the roast potatoes. But the FastDiet seems to be different: men have been adopting it in droves. They appear to like the clarity of the 600-calorie, twice-a-week rule. On a Fast Day, many men choose to eat nothing at all (staying hydrated, of course) until the evening, when they'll sit down to a decent meal. That's where this chapter comes in. Man food. Under 600 calories. Done.

SIMPLE SEARED SIRLOIN AND FIVE QUICK ACCOMPANIMENTS . . .

183 CALORIES PER PORTION FOR A PLAIN STEAK

Serves 1

7 ounces/200g sirloin steak, trimmed of visible fat
Olive oil

Salt and freshly ground black pepper

Heat a grill pan until searingly hot. Rub the steak with a little oil, season well, and sear for 2 to 3 minutes on each side, or until cooked to your liking. Let rest and prepare with one of the following:

. . . arugula and watercress with horseradish cream

+80 CALORIES PER PORTION

2 tablespoons low-fat crème fraîche
1 teaspoon horseradish sauce

Juice of ½ lemon
Snipped fresh chives
Small bunch of arugula and watercress

Combine the ingredients and serve alongside the steak and a generous mass of arugula and watercress. If you have calories to spare, add a scant crumble of blue cheese (+45 calories per tablespoon).

. . . pepper sauce

+104 CALORIES PER PORTION

Cooking spray
2 small shallots, finely chopped
Scant ½ cup/100ml chicken stock
1 tablespoon low-fat garlic soft
 cheese

1 tablespoon low-fat crème
 fraîche
1 teaspoon coarsely crushed
 peppercorns

After removing the steak and setting aside to rest, coat the grill pan with cooking spray and sauté the shallots until softened. Lower the heat and add the stock, cheese, crème fraîche, and peppercorns and stir well with a spatula. Simmer for 2 minutes until the sauce is slightly thickened, then drizzle on the steak. Curly kale would be good on the side.

. . . chili dipping sauce and bok choy

+109 CALORIES PER PORTION

1 red chile, seeded and very
 finely chopped
1 garlic clove, crushed
1 teaspoon sugar
1 tablespoon Thai fish sauce

1 tablespoon lime juice
1 tablespoon chopped mint
5 ounces/150g bok choy, sliced
 into strips

Mix the sauce ingredients in a bowl. Steam the bok choy for 3 minutes and drain well. Slice the steak thinly, serve on top of the bok choy, and drizzle with the dipping sauce.

... herb dressing

Handful of fresh tarragon leaves, chopped
Handful of fresh basil leaves, torn
1 tablespoon olive oil
½ tablespoon lemon juice
½ tablespoon white wine
½ teaspoon sugar

Combine the ingredients well and pour over the steak and your chosen vegetable. Fine green beans or lightly steamed asparagus would be ideal.

... baked tomatoes and olives

+140 CALORIES PER PORTION

8 to 10 cherry tomatoes
½ tablespoon olive oil
Pinch of red pepper flakes
Salt and freshly ground black pepper
4 black olives, halved and pitted

Preheat the oven to 400°F. Place the ingredients in a small ovenproof dish and bake for 15 to 20 minutes. Serve alongside the steak, spooning with the tomato juices.

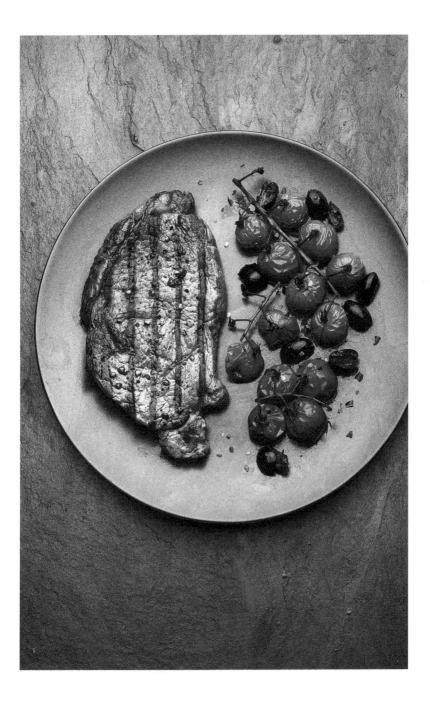

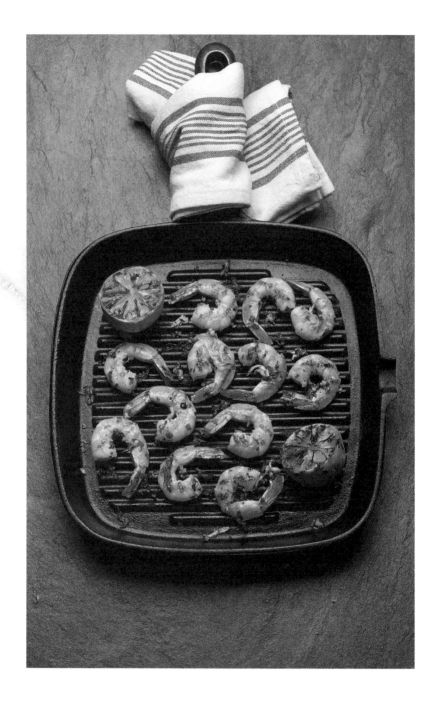

GARLIC AND PARSLEY SHRIMP

215 CALORIES PER PORTION

Serves 2

Shrimp are a FastDieter's faithful friend—under 60 calories per 3½ ounces/100g, easy to haul from the freezer, and a bolt of protein with no carbs and barely any fat.

10 to 15 raw large shrimp (about 7 ounces/200g), peeled, tails intact
3 small garlic cloves, crushed
1 tablespoon olive oil
1 tablespoon lemon juice
1 tablespoon finely chopped fresh flat-leaf parsley
Salt and cracked black pepper
Lemon wedges, for serving

Combine all the ingredients in a bowl and rest in the fridge to allow the flavors to develop. Heat a grill pan to medium heat and cook the shrimp for 2 to 3 minutes, turning once—they should be pink but still juicy. Serve with lemon wedges and a substantial bowl of lemon-dressed herb salad.

FAST DAY TIP: Grilling seals in flavor while allowing any excess cooking fat to run off along the ridges of the pan. Look for a heavy grill pan with well-spaced ridges; when cooking, don't be tempted to move the fish or meat around too much, even if it appears to be sticking. Have faith: once cooked, it will unstick itself.

● Goes well with Chunky Cumin Coleslaw, page 114 (+74 calories per portion).

TEN-MINUTE JUMBO SHRIMP CURRY

222 CALORIES PER PORTION

Serves 2

Shrimp are one of the speediest fridge-to-plate options around. This really does take ten minutes start to end—if you eat it slowly and with relish, it should take longer to consume than to cook.

2 tablespoons medium or hot curry paste
2 tablespoons cold water
1 medium red onion, finely sliced
1 medium red bell pepper, seeded and sliced
1 red chile, seeded and finely chopped
1 tablespoon mango chutney
3 large ripe tomatoes, cored and coarsely chopped
⅔ cup/150ml low-fat coconut milk
7 ounces/200g cooked or raw jumbo shrimp
3½ ounces/100g baby spinach leaves
Lime juice and fresh cilantro leaves, for serving

Heat a large pan and add curry paste, water, onion, bell pepper, and chile and cook for 4 minutes, until softened, stirring well. Add the chutney, tomatoes, and coconut milk and simmer for 3 minutes. Add the shrimp and spinach, cook until the shrimp are pink and the spinach has just wilted, about 3 minutes. Serve with a squeeze of lime and the cilantro leaves.

OPTIONAL EXTRAS: Store-bought low-calorie naan bread would add 120 calories.

BEEF CHILI STIR-FRY

230 CALORIES PER PORTION

Serves 4

1 teaspoon olive oil

5 scallions, sliced on the diagonal

14 ounces/400g lean ground beef

1¼-inch/3cm piece fresh ginger, peeled and grated

3 garlic cloves, crushed

1 teaspoon Chinese five-spice powder

½ teaspoon chili powder

1 cup/250ml beef stock or boiling water and beef bouillon cube

3 tablespoons soy sauce

5 ounces/150g snow peas

5 ounces/150g sugar snap peas

1 red chile, seeded and finely sliced, for serving

Heat the oil in a large wok and stir-fry the scallions for 1 minute. Then add the beef and cook for another 5 to 6 minutes, or until browned. Add the ginger, garlic, five-spice and chili powders and sauté for a few minutes more. Add the stock and soy sauce, bring to a boil, stirring occasionally, and simmer for 5 minutes. Add the snow peas and sugar snaps and cook until the vegetables are just done. Serve topped with red chile slices.

OPTIONAL EXTRAS: Add 3½ ounces/100g chopped oyster or shiitake mushrooms along with the snow peas to bulk out the dish at negligible calorie cost.

● Goes well with fresh egg noodles, if your calorie count allows (+130 calories per 3½ ounces/100g).

LAMB BURGERS WITH HOT TOMATO SAUCE

234 CALORIES PER PORTION

Serves 4

I love these fiery burgers. By all means, use leftover lamb—but make sure that you're using the least fatty meat: The fat in lamb can quickly bust your calorie count.

For the sauce
- 1 cup/240g canned crushed tomatoes
- 1 tablespoon tomato paste
- 1 red chile, halved (seeded to taste)
- 1 teaspoon dried oregano
- ½ teaspoon sugar

For the burgers
- 14 ounces/400g lean cooked lamb, ground
- 1 small onion, finely chopped
- 2 garlic cloves, crushed
- 1 tablespoon harissa paste
- 2 tablespoons/30g bread crumbs
- 2 large eggs, beaten
- Salt and freshly ground black pepper
- Cooking spray
- 4 tablespoons low-fat plain yogurt and chopped fresh cilantro, for serving

Simmer the sauce ingredients in a small saucepan for 20 minutes and set aside. In a large bowl, mix the lamb, onion, garlic, harissa paste, bread crumbs, and eggs. Season with salt and pepper. Divide into 8 patties. Spray a large frying pan with oil and sauté the burgers on medium heat until browned. Lower the heat and cook for another 5 to 10 minutes, until cooked, turning once. Serve with the hot sauce on the side, plus a cooling tablespoon of yogurt, cilantro, and a lemon-dressed side salad.

OPTIONAL EXTRAS: Add fresh mint, dried rosemary and thyme, or chopped capers to the burger mix.

● Goes well with Yellow Squash and Almond Salad, page 125 (+253 calories per porton).

LAMB CHOPS WITH PEAS

263 CALORIES PER PORTION

Serves 4

1 teaspoon olive oil
2 tablespoons balsamic vinegar
2 teaspoons fresh thyme leaves
Salt and freshly ground black
  pepper
4 shoulder lamb chops (about
  3½ ounces/100g each),
  trimmed of excess fat

1 pound/450g frozen peas
2 tablespoons/30g butter
Handful of fresh mint leaves,
  chopped
Squeeze of lemon
Sea salt

Combine the oil, vinegar, thyme, salt, and pepper in a bowl or plastic bag. Add the lamb chops and coat well, then leave for up to a day in the fridge to marinate. Heat a grill pan until very hot, and sear the lamb for 1 to 2 minutes on each side, or until done to your liking. Set aside to rest. Meanwhile, cook the peas, strain, and then blend them with butter, mint, lemon, and sea salt. Serve with the lamb.

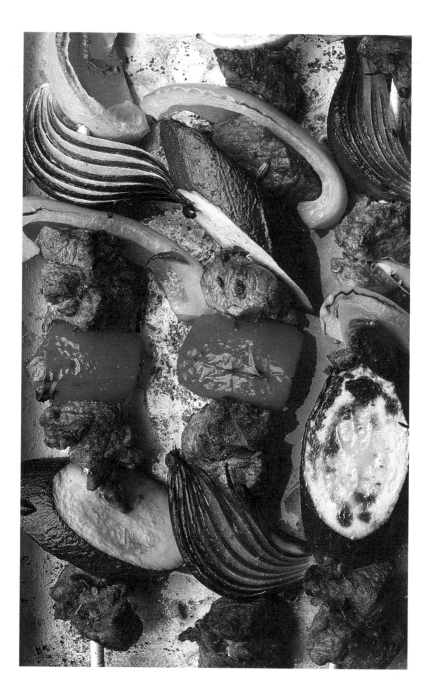

EASY LAMB KEBABS

267 CALORIES PER PORTION

Serves 4, making 8 kebabs

For the marinade
2 teaspoons ground cumin
2 teaspoons ground coriander
½ teaspoon red pepper flakes
1 teaspoon fennel seeds
1 tablespoon fresh thyme leaves
Zest and juice of 1 lemon
1 garlic clove, crushed
1 tablespoon olive oil
Salt and freshly ground black
   pepper

For the kebabs
1½ pounds/700g lean lamb,
   trimmed of excess fat and
   cubed
2 medium red onions, cut into
   wedges (keep the root intact)
2 medium zucchini, cut into
   1¼-inch/3cm rounds
2 medium yellow bell peppers,
   seeded and cut into chunks
2 medium red bell peppers,
   seeded and cut into chunks
1 lemon, cut into 8 wedges

Combine the marinade ingredients in a bowl or plastic bag. Add the lamb and leave to marinate in the fridge for at least an hour, or preferably overnight. Prepare the kebabs on metal skewers, alternating meat and veggies and ending with a lemon wedge. Brush with any remaining marinade. Cook on a hot grill for 6 to 8 minutes, turning occasionally and spooning over any excess marinade. These are great barbecued, of course, or cooked on a hot grill pan.

● Goes well with Chunky Cumin Coleslaw, page 114 (+74 calories per portion).

OPTIONAL EXTRA: Add firm mushrooms or eggplant cubes to boost your veggie intake.

HUEVOS RANCHEROS

Serves 1

Add a little Mexican twist to suppertime (or to breakfast, for that matter, if you're looking for something substantial). Eggs are a prime Fast Day food, and this way of serving them is a welcome break from the usual suspects.

1 teaspoon olive oil
2 scallions, finely chopped
1 medium red bell pepper, seeded and sliced
¼ teaspoon red pepper flakes
¾ cup/200g canned diced tomatoes

1 teaspoon balsamic vinegar
Salt and freshly ground black pepper
2 large eggs
Handful of fresh flat-leaf parsley, coarsely chopped

Heat the oil in a small frying pan and sauté the scallions, bell pepper, and red pepper flakes for 3 minutes. Add the tomatoes and vinegar. Season, stir, and simmer for 5 minutes. Make two dips in the sauce and crack an egg into each. Continue cooking until the whites have begun to set, then cover and cook until they are completely set, but the yolks are still runny. Sprinkle with parsley and serve.

OPTIONAL EXTRA: Serve with avocado (+150 calories per half), chili sauce (25 calories per tablespoon) and a whole-grain tortilla (about 90 calories) if you want the full enchilada. The total calorie count per portion would then be 548.

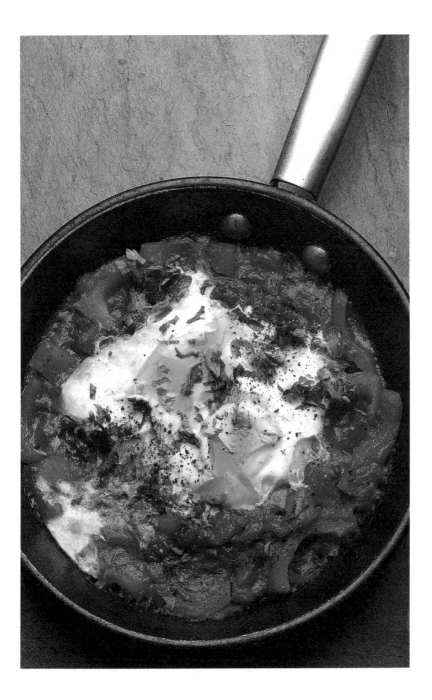

TURKEY KOFTE WITH TZATZIKI AND WARM PITA

310 CALORIES PER PORTION

Serves 4

Using ground turkey rather than the traditional lamb really lowers the calorie count of these tasty kofte.

For the kofte
1 pound/450g lean ground turkey
3 garlic cloves, crushed
1 teaspoon ground cumin
1 teaspoon ground coriander
½ teaspoon red pepper flakes
½ teaspoon ground allspice
Zest of ½ lemon
2 tablespoons fresh mint, chopped
2 tablespoons chopped fresh flat-leaf parsley
Salt and black pepper
Cooking spray

For the tzatziki
½ cup/100g low-fat plain yogurt
1 garlic clove, crushed
½ small cucumber, peeled, seeded, and diced
Fresh cilantro leaves, chopped
Fresh mint leaves, chopped
Squeeze of lemon
Salt and freshly ground black pepper

4 whole wheat pitas (6½-inch diameter)
2 teaspoons cumin seeds, toasted in a small frying pan

Combine the kofte ingredients in a large bowl until evenly mixed, then shape around eight metal or pre-soaked wooden skewers. Chill for a ½ hour, spray with a little oil, then place on a lightly oiled, foil-lined baking sheet and grill on medium-high heat for 10 to 12 minutes, turning once. Combine the tzatziki ingredients in a small bowl. Place the kofte in warm pitas, drizzle with the tzatziki, and scatter with the cumin seeds.

FAST DAY TIP: If you have the kofte and tzatziki without the pita, the calorie count dives to 173 per portion. Kofte freeze well so it's worth making in double quantities.

THREE-PEPPER FAJITA SALAD

262 CALORIES PER PORTION

Serves 4

One of the fundamentals for successful Fast Day cooking is keeping your taste buds amused. Rather than relying on bland, boring foods, go instead for chile fire and tantalizing texture. You'll get exactly that from this fabulous fajita salad.

3 teaspoons extra-virgin olive oil
2 tablespoons water
1 large sweet onion, thinly sliced
3 medium bell peppers (green, red, yellow, orange), seeded and cut into ½- to ¾-inch squares

¾ teaspoon dried oregano
1½ teaspoons chili powder
1 teaspoon salt
½ teaspoon black pepper
1 pound/450g flank steak
1 lime, halved
6 cups shredded romaine lettuce

In a large nonstick skillet, heat 2 teaspoons of the oil and the water over medium heat. Add the onion and bell peppers, sprinkle with the oregano, ¾ teaspoon of the chili powder, ½ teaspoon of the salt, and ¼ teaspoon of the black pepper. Cover and cook until tender and wilted, 7 to 9 minutes. Let stand, uncovered, until cooled to warm or room temperature. Rub the flank steak on both sides with the remaining ¾ teaspoon chili powder, ½ teaspoon salt, and ¼ teaspoon black pepper. Preheat a grill pan over medium heat. Add the remaining 1 teaspoon oil. Grill the steak for about 5 minutes per side for medium-rare (about 1 minute more per side for medium). Squeeze one lime half over the steak. Let rest for 6 minutes before thinly slicing against the grain and then cutting into bite-size pieces. In a large salad bowl, toss together the meat (and any meat juices) and onion mixture (and all pan juices). Squeeze in the remaining lime juice and toss well with the lettuce.

● You can cook the onion and pepper mixture well ahead.

OPTIONAL EXTRA: You can add 1 tablespoon crumbled baked tortilla chips to each salad serving for about 60 calories.

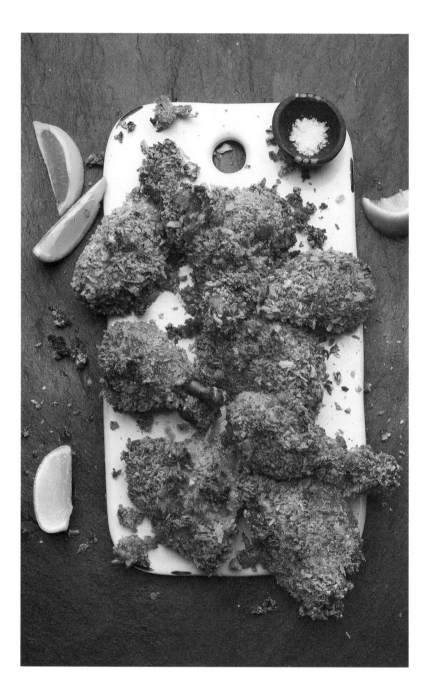

PANKO "FRIED" CHICKEN

335 CALORIES PER PORTION

Serves 4

Not fried, of course. But the panko—a Japanese-style bread crumb that doesn't absorb as much fat as traditional crumbs—delivers a crispy-crunchy coating which is just as good to eat.

1 cup/250ml buttermilk	4 skinless chicken drumsticks
Salt and freshly ground black	4 skinless chicken thighs
pepper	3½ ounces/100g panko
1 teaspoon ground ginger	bread crumbs
1 teaspoon ground turmeric	Cooking spray
2 teaspoons ground coriander	Lemon wedges, for serving
2 teaspoons paprika	

Combine the buttermilk, salt, pepper, ginger, turmeric, 1 teaspoon of the coriander, and 1 teaspoon of the paprika in a large bowl. Add the chicken and toss. Leave to marinate in the fridge for 3 hours, or overnight if possible. Preheat the oven to 375°F. Put the panko in a bowl and season with the remaining 1 teaspoon coriander, the remaining 1 teaspoon paprika, the salt, and pepper. Coat each chicken piece in seasoned panko. Place on a baking sheet lined with nonstick foil, or sprayed with a little cooking oil. Bake for 35 to 40 minutes, or until golden brown and cooked through, turning once if necessary. Serve with lemon wedges and a simple green salad.

● Goes well with Big Baked Beans, page 133 (+265 calories per portion).

CHEAT'S TIP: If buttermilk is hard to find, substitute with 1 cup/200g low-fat plain yogurt mixed with ¼ cup/50ml low-fat milk.

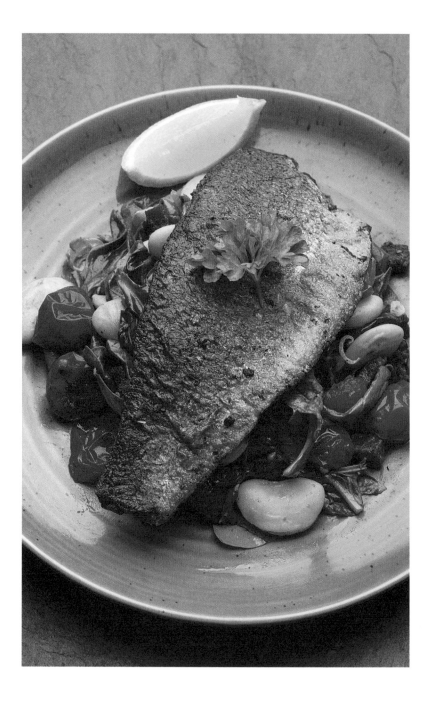

SEA BASS WITH TOMATO, CHORIZO, AND BUTTER BEANS

385 CALORIES PER PORTION

Serves 2

This is one of my all-time great standby suppers, particularly if I'm having friends over to eat. It looks great, tastes utterly delicious, and is surprisingly foolproof.

2 sea bass fillets, about 7 ounces/200g each
Salt and freshly ground black pepper
2 tablespoons/30g coarsely chopped chorizo sausage
10 cherry tomatoes, halved
1 garlic clove, crushed
1 teaspoon dried parsley
1 (14-ounce/400g) can butter beans
1 (9-ounce/250g) bag baby spinach
Squeeze of lemon
Cooking spray
Chopped fresh parsley and lemon wedges, for serving

Season the fillets and score the skin to prevent it from curling during cooking. Sauté the chorizo in a dry pan until it releases its oil, flavor, and color. Add the tomatoes, garlic, and dried parsley and cook for 2 minutes, until the tomatoes soften. Add the butter beans and simmer for 2 minutes so they are heated through. Add the spinach and lemon juice for the final minute of cooking, then remove from the pan and set aside. Spray a little cooking oil in the same pan and when hot, sear the sea bass skin side down for 3 minutes, or until crisp. Flip it over and cook on the other side for 2 minutes. Place on a mound of the warm butter bean mixture and serve with parsley and lemon wedges.

OPTIONAL EXTRA: Add 1 teaspoon of fennel seeds along with the tomatoes and parsley. Or 6 black olives, halved and pitted, for extra depth (+30 calories).

● Try sea bream or red mullet fillets as an alternative to sea bass.

BUFFALO CHICKEN BURGERS WITH BLUE CHEESE AND CELERY RELISH

273 CALORIES PER PORTION

Serves 4

Chicken and blue cheese—a marriage made in heaven. But on a Fast Day? Why not? This dish follows the FastDiet strategy of using lean protein and plenty of full-on flavor. The pita really does add to the equation, but if you're up against your quota for the day, drop it and save 80 calories.

1¼ pounds/565g ground chicken
1 tablespoon plus ¼ teaspoon
    Louisiana-style hot sauce
5 scallions, white and pale green
    parts chopped, dark greens
    reserved
½ teaspoon salt
1 large celery stalk, minced
½ teaspoon grated lemon zest

2 teaspoons lemon juice
Cooking spray
1 ounce crumbled blue cheese
¼ cup/50g nonfat Greek yogurt
Freshly ground black pepper
4 whole wheat pitas (4-inch
    diameter), split and lightly
    toasted

In a large bowl, combine the chicken, the 1 tablespoon hot sauce, the scallions, and salt. With wet hands, form into 4 patties 3½ inches across. In a small bowl, combine the celery, lemon zest and juice, and the remaining ¼ teaspoon hot sauce. Slice 2 tablespoons of the scallion dark greens and add to the bowl. Preheat a stovetop grill pan over medium-high heat. Coat generously with cooking spray and add the burgers. Cook without turning for 3 minutes. Flip and cook for 4 minutes. Flip again (and orient the patties so you get different grill marks) and cook for 2 minutes. Flip a final time, turn off the heat, and let the burgers sit for 1 minute. In a small bowl, use a fork to mash together the blue cheese, yogurt, and a couple grinds of pepper until smoothish. Serve the burgers on the pita with celery relish and blue cheese topping.

● Goes well with steamed asparagus and Chunky Cumin Coleslaw, page 114 (+74 calories per portion).

MAN FOOD FOR A FAST DAY

BREAKFAST: If in doubt, eat an egg. A two-egg chile and scallion omelet has 180 calories; scrambled eggs with 2½ ounces/80g smoked salmon have 300. If you need carbs to start the day, go for oatmeal—perhaps with chopped pear and cinnamon (286 calories).

SUPPER: Max out the vegetables and minimize the carbs. You need protein, too; white fish, shellfish, and chicken are best. Add flavor rather than calories with lemon, cumin, chile, lime, ginger, onion. . . . You can have curry, but if you're short of calories, go for fish or shrimp instead of meat. Dahl is an ideal choice, see page 131.

TAKEOUT: Sashimi boxes are great for a hit of protein (avoid the sushi rice). Soup is good, too—but go for the clear, veggie-laden stocks, not the heavier, meaty, cheesy alternatives.

SNACKS: Not really part of the plan. But if you must, have a handful of almonds, or strawberries, carrots and hummus, or an apple. Include the calorie count in your quota.

DRINKING: Stay hydrated. Alcohol is "empty" calories (an 18½ ounce/550ml beer racks up 250 calories). If you must, vodka has the fewest calories; soda and lemon juice are the best mixers; orange juice doubles the calorie count of a vodka shot.

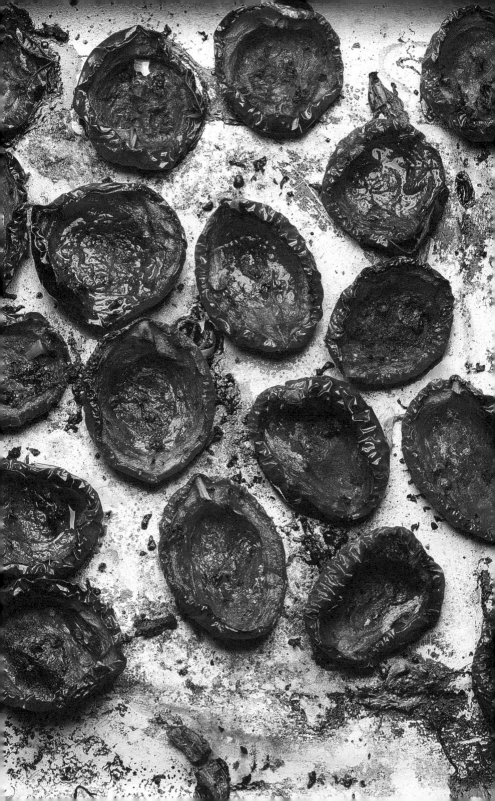

Simple Sides

Ideal Alone, or to Partner a Supper of Chicken or Fish

Plenty of people simply eat grilled fish or chicken on a Fast Day. Here's how to pep up the plate with easy, healthy sides and salads. You may, of course, choose to make these dishes the main event; many are full of protein and need no further fuss.

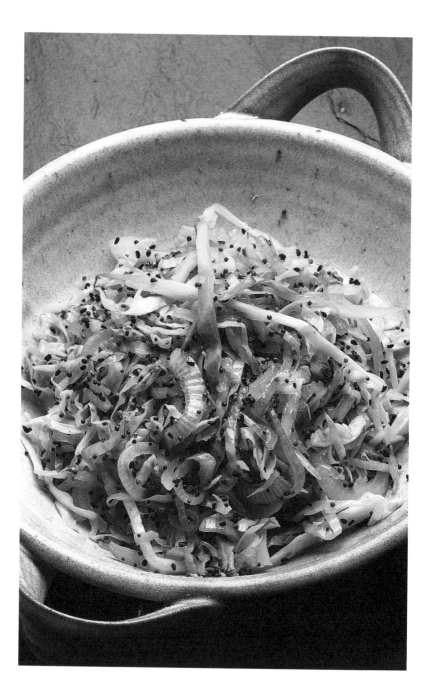

SPRING CABBAGE WITH MUSTARD SEEDS

27 CALORIES PER PORTION

Serves 4 as a side dish

1 tablespoon mustard seeds

1 teaspoon olive oil

1 small onion, finely sliced

1 garlic clove, crushed

1 tablespoon grated fresh ginger

1 pound/450g spring cabbage,
  shredded

2 tablespoons water

Toast the mustard seeds until they start to pop. Add the oil, then sauté the onion, garlic, and ginger until golden. Add the cabbage and stir to coat with the spices, add the water and cook for 5 minutes, until tender. Season and serve.

CAULIFLOWER "COUSCOUS"

36 CALORIES PER PORTION

Serves 4 as a side dish

1 large cauliflower, divided
  into florets
¼ cup water
Salt and freshly ground black pepper

Place the cauliflower in a food processor and pulse until it resembles bread crumbs. Bring the water to a simmer in a large frying pan and add the cauliflower. Steam gently for 3 to 4 minutes, season and serve.

OPTIONAL EXTRAS: This works with any number of additions. Try adding 1 teaspoon chopped fresh rosemary or thyme, 2 finely sliced scallions, and 2 teaspoons lemon zest during the cooking time. Or add 1 tablespoon each of finely chopped celery, raisins (+33 calories), and chopped apple (+15 calories) once cooked. Walnuts (+50 calories), pine nuts (+58 calories), orange zest, dried cranberries (+26 calories), and pomegranate seeds (+9 calories) are good additions too—or a simple handful of chopped cilantro for color and flavor.

● Goes well with any tagine, pages 64–67.

LEMON-PEPPER BROCCOLI WITH COCONUT OIL

64 CALORIES PER PORTION

Serves 4 as a side dish

If all the goodness in the world were to be condensed into one small package, it would probably look a lot like broccoli. Broccoli is a fine source of vitamins, including K (useful to guard against osteoporosis)—and it's easy to "dress it up" to make it feel like a treat on the plate. The lemon here gives it a welcome tang, and the dash of oil will help release its fat-soluble vitamins.

1 medium bunch (2 heads) broccoli
Grated zest of 1 lemon
1 tablespoon lemon juice
1 tablespoon coconut oil
½ teaspoon coarse (kosher) salt
½ teaspoon black pepper

Cut the broccoli tops into small florets. Thinly slice the stems crosswise (peel them first if the skin seems especially thick or woody). In a vegetable steamer, steam the broccoli until tender, 8 to 10 minutes (depending on the thickness and toughness of the stem pieces. Meanwhile, put the lemon zest and juice, oil, salt, and pepper in a large bowl. Add the hot broccoli to the bowl and toss well to coat.

● You could also make this with broccolini or broccoli rabe. The steaming time will be shorter for these smaller broccolis. For the broccoli rabe, add a little grated garlic, too.

CHUNKY CUMIN COLESLAW

74 CALORIES PER PORTION

Serves 4 as a side dish

½ medium white cabbage, coarsely shredded
2 medium carrots, peeled and grated
1 medium apple, peeled and grated
2 teaspoons cumin seeds, toasted in a small frying pan

¼ teaspoon ground cumin
2 tablespoons low-fat plain yogurt
2 teaspoons lemon juice
1 tablespoon golden raisins
Salt and freshly ground black pepper

Combine all the ingredients and serve.

OPTIONAL EXTRA: Include shredded celery root or fennel, or a handful of walnuts (+50 calories) for added crunch and protein.

● Goes well with Easy Lamb Kebabs, page 97 (+267 calories per portion).

SPICED RED CABBAGE
WITH APPLES

79 CALORIES PER PORTION

Serves 6 as a side dish

Cooking spray
1 medium onion, finely diced
2 medium apples, peeled and
   cubed
1 medium red cabbage,
   quartered and finely sliced
3 tablespoons red wine vinegar
1 bay leaf
1 cinnamon stick

½ teaspoon ground ginger
½ teaspoon ground coriander
1 whole clove
1 cardamom pod
1 cup/250ml natural apple juice
1 tablespoon honey
Salt and freshly ground black
   pepper

Heat a pan coated with cooking spray. Add the onion and cook until softened. Add the apples and cook for 3 minutes, stirring gently. Add the cabbage, vinegar, bay leaf, spices, apple juice, and honey. Stir, cover, and simmer for 25 minutes, or until the cabbage is tender. Season and serve.

● Goes well with Hot Paprika Goulash, page 23 (+275 calories per portion).

● This is even better the next day, and it freezes well.

CELERY ROOT REMOULADE

92 CALORIES PER PORTION

Serves 4 as a side dish

14 ounces/400g celery root, peeled

For the dressing
2 tablespoons lemon juice
2 tablespoons mayonnaise
2 tablespoons low-fat plain yogurt
2 tablespoons Dijon mustard
Salt and freshly ground black pepper

Use a food processor or a mandoline to julienne the celery root into fine matchsticks. Do not grate as it will become too mushy. Toss in the combined dressing ingredients and serve.

OPTIONAL EXTRAS: Thinly sliced fennel and celery can be added to the celery root. Swap the lemon juice for orange juice and add grated carrot as an alternative. Or add aniseed and finely chopped tarragon.

● Goes well with smoked trout.

TABBOULEH

123 CALORIES PER PORTION

Serves 4 as a side dish

Tabbouleh is a parsley salad, not a bulgar salad; herbs should predominate. As an alternative to bulgar, you could use buckwheat (it is also lower GI).

2½ ounces/75g bulgar wheat
1 teaspoon ground allspice
1 teaspoon ground cinnamon
1 teaspoon ground coriander
4 medium ripe tomatoes, cored and chopped
4 scallions, finely sliced
Juice of 2 lemons
½ large bunch of fresh flat-leaf parsley, finely chopped
½ large bunch of fresh mint, finely chopped
2 tablespoons pomegranate seeds
2 tablespoons olive oil
Salt and freshly ground black pepper

Soak the bulgar wheat and spices in almost-boiling water and set aside until softened, about 20 minutes. Fluff up with a fork, then add the tomatoes, scallions, and lemon juice. Stir well, add the herbs, pomegranate seeds, and oil. Season and serve.

● If you prefer the tomatoes peeled, immerse them in boiling water for 2 to 3 minutes and then peel.

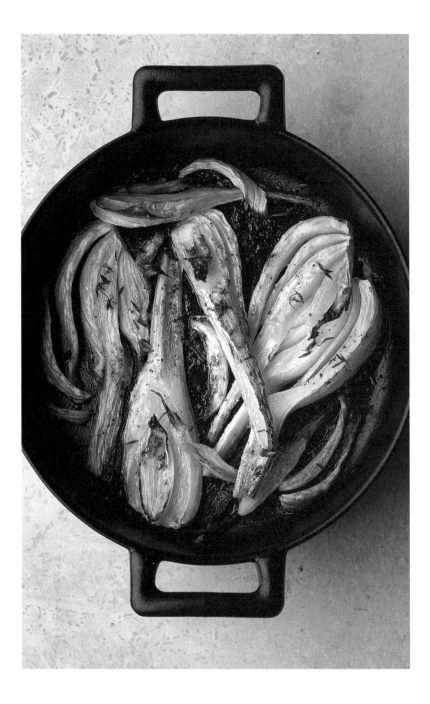

BAKED FENNEL WITH PARMESAN AND THYME

123 CALORIES PER PORTION

Serves 2 as a side dish

2 medium fennel bulbs, trimmed
   and quartered
1 tablespoon olive oil
1 tablespoon lemon juice
Salt and freshly ground black
   pepper

2 tablespoons/30g grated
   Parmesan cheese
1 teaspoon dried thyme, or 1
   tablespoon fresh thyme leaves

Preheat the oven to 400°F. Place the fennel in a small roasting pan, coat with oil and lemon juice, then season and scatter with the Parmesan and thyme. Cover with foil and bake for 30 minutes, until soft.

● Goes well with Dijon chicken, page 42 (+210 calories per portion).

● Try this with leeks or chicory, or a mix of both.

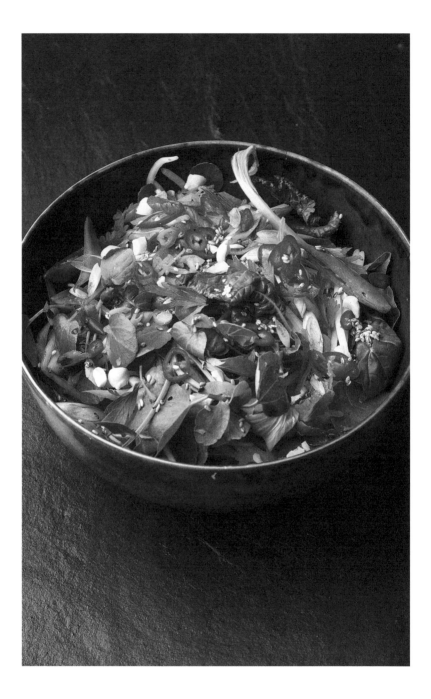

ASIAN SESAME SALAD

133 CALORIES PER PORTION

Serves 2 as a side dish

For the salad
1 bok choy, sliced into ribbons
Chinese cabbage or Savoy
  cabbage, leaves torn
Handful of bean sprouts
Handful of snow peas, sliced on
  diagonal
Handful of watercress
1 medium carrot, peeled and
  grated
1 scallion, sliced on the diagonal
Handful of fresh cilantro,
  chopped

For the dressing
1 teaspoon palm sugar
1 teaspoon toasted sesame oil
1 teaspoon soy sauce
½ tablespoon Thai fish sauce
Juice of 1 lime
1 red chile, finely sliced
  (optional)
10 cashews, coarsely chopped,
  and 3 teaspoons sesame
  seeds, toasted, for serving

Assemble the salad ingredients, toss with the combined dressing ingredients, and serve topped with cashews, sesame seeds, and fresh chile, if desired.

● Goes well with No-Fuss Fish with Chili Dressing, page 45 (+175 calories per portion).

INSTEAD OF MASHED POTATOES. . .

. . . cauliflower mash

142 CALORIES PER PORTION

Serves 2 as a side dish

1 tablespoon olive oil
1 small onion, finely chopped
1 garlic clove, crushed
1 medium leek, finely sliced
½ teaspoon ground turmeric
Salt and freshly ground black
  pepper

1 small cauliflower, divided into
  florets
3 tablespoons/50ml vegetable
  stock or boiling water with half
  a vegetable bouillon cube
Squeeze of lemon

In a large pan, heat the oil and sauté the onion, garlic, and leek until softened. Add the turmeric, season with salt and pepper, and cook for 1 minute. Add the cauliflower and stir well to coat with the spiced onion mixture. Add the stock, cover, and cook gently for 10 minutes. Puree with a hand blender, or mash well. Add lemon juice and serve.

. . . cannellini bean mash

183 CALORIES PER PORTION

Serves 2 as a side dish

1 (14-ounce/400g) can
  cannellini beans, rinsed
  and drained
2 tablespoons 1% low-fat milk

1 vegetable or chicken
  bouillon cube
1 tablespoon olive oil
Salt and cracked black pepper

Heat all the ingredients, then puree with a hand blender or mash well. Return briefly to the heat if you like your mash piping hot. Season with salt and plenty of pepper and serve.

OPTIONAL EXTRA: Add red pepper flakes, chopped fresh herbs (sage would be good), and a squeeze of lime to the bean mash for extra zing.

FAST DAY TIP: This is very good served cold as a dip for raw veggies; loosen with a little low-fat yogurt and garnish with parsley, a squeeze of lemon, and paprika.

... sweet potato and carrot mash

183 CALORIES PER PORTION

Serves 2 as a side dish

10½ ounces/300g carrots, peeled and chopped
10½ ounces/300g sweet potatoes, peeled and chopped
2 garlic cloves, crushed
1 teaspoon cumin seeds, toasted in a small frying pan

1 tablespoon/15g butter
Salt and freshly ground black pepper
2 or 3 tablespoons 1% low-fat milk (optional)

Place the carrots, sweet potatoes, and garlic in a large saucepan of salted water, bring to a boil, then cook until tender, 12 to 15 minutes. Drain, add the cumin seeds, butter, and seasoning. Coarsely mash, adding a dash of milk if you prefer a looser consistency, then serve.

FAST DAY TIP: If you can't bear to go without mashed potatoes, cut the calories by using low-fat crème fraîche rather than butter. Or mix with sliced steamed leeks, or add a handful of watercress leaves after mashing, which will wilt prettily in the heat.

THREE WARM SALADS . . .

. . . spiced brown lentils with mint

171 CALORIES PER PORTION

Serves 2 as a side dish

7 ounces/200g brown
lentils, rinsed
1 bay leaf
Cooking spray
1 medium red onion, finely
chopped
1 garlic clove, crushed
½ teaspoon ground cumin
½ teaspoon paprika
2 cardamom pods

For the dressing
Generous handful of fresh
mint leaves, chopped
1 tablespoon olive oil
1 tablespoon red wine vinegar
Salt and freshly ground black
pepper
2 scallions, finely sliced,
for garnish

Place the lentils in a saucepan with the bay leaf, cover with water, and simmer for 15 to 20 minutes, or until tender. Spray a small frying pan with oil and sauté the onion, garlic, and spices for 3 minutes, until the onion starts to soften. Remove the cardamom pods. In a small bowl, combine the dressing ingredients and whisk well. Drain the lentils, remove the bay leaf, then combine with the onion mixture and drizzle with the mint vinaigrette. Serve warm, topped with scallions.

. . . yellow squash and almond

253 CALORIES PER PORTION

Serves 2 as a side dish

For the dressing
1 tablespoon olive oil
1 tablespoon balsamic vinegar
1 tablespoon lemon juice
1 teaspoon honey
½ teaspoon cumin seeds,
    toasted in a small frying pan
Salt and freshly ground black
    pepper

For the salad
Cooking spray
9 ounces/250g young yellow
    squash, sliced lengthwise into
    ⅛-inch/2mm thick ribbons
1¾ ounces/50g whole blanched
    almonds
2½ ounces/75g baby herb
    salad leaves

Mix the dressing ingredients and set aside. Heat the oil in a grill pan and sauté the squash and almonds for 2 to 3 minutes. Combine the squash, almonds, and salad leaves, and add the dressing. Season and serve.

OPTIONAL EXTRA: Add a crumble of feta for tang and extra protein (+25 calories per tablespoon).

... green lentil, orange, and hazelnut

358 CALORIES PER PORTION

Serves 2

For the dressing
1 tablespoon olive oil
1 tablespoon balsamic vinegar
2 tablespoons orange juice
1 garlic clove, very finely
  chopped
Salt and freshly ground black
  pepper

For the salad
1 (9-ounce/250g) bag ready-to-eat
  green lentils
½ medium red onion, finely
  chopped
1 large carrot, peeled and grated
2 tablespoons/30g roasted
  chopped hazelnuts
Generous handful of fresh curly
  parsley, chopped
1 tablespoon grated orange zest,
  for serving

Combine the oil, vinegar, orange juice, garlic, salt, and pepper in a small bowl. Microwave the lentils in the bag for 1 minute, then add the lentils to the bowl and stir in the onion, carrot, hazelnuts, and parsley. Mix well and serve at room temperature, scattered with orange zest.

OPTIONAL EXTRA: Top each portion with ¼ cup/40g cubed marinated tofu for a more substantial supper (+60 calories). As an alternative, replace the carrot with a handful of chopped Homemade Oven-Dried Tomatoes, page 145 (+20 calories for 3½ ounces/100g).

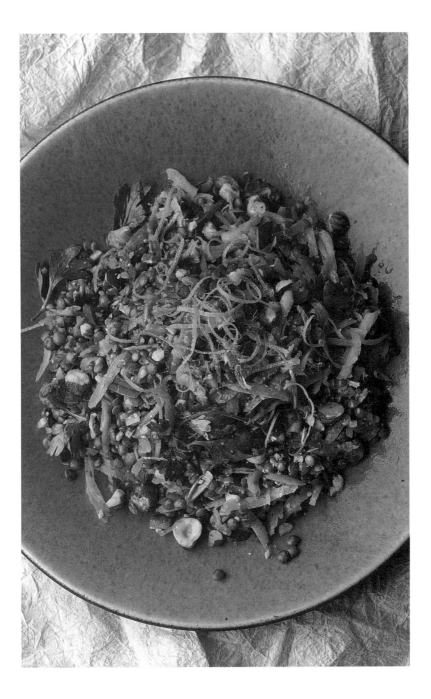

HOW TO STUFF A MUSHROOM. . .

Eating mushrooms in place of red meat can significantly slash your calorie intake so swap them when you can. A big meadow mushroom works well as transport for veggies and punchy flavors, and all of these recipes will make a filling midweek supper. If you can't get a big meadow mushroom, two smaller portobello mushrooms would work just as well.

. . . with spinach, chiles, and cheese

173 CALORIES PER PORTION

Serves 1

Cooking spray
½ small red onion, finely chopped
1 small garlic clove, finely chopped
Pinch of red pepper flakes
3½ ounces/100g baby spinach
 leaves

1 large meadow mushroom,
 cleaned and trimmed
1 teaspoon olive oil
1 tablespoon bread crumbs
1 tablespoon grated Parmesan
 cheese

Preheat the oven to 350°F. Heat a small pan, coat with cooking spray, and sauté the onion, garlic, and red pepper flakes until softened. Add the spinach, stir, and cook gently until wilted. Drizzle the mushroom with oil and season well. Spoon the spinach mixture into the cap. Sprinkle with bread crumbs and Parmesan, then bake for 15 to 20 minutes and serve.

... with goat cheese and walnuts

275 CALORIES PER PORTION

Serves 1

1 large meadow mushroom,
  cleaned and trimmed, stem
  removed and chopped
1¾ ounces/50g soft goat cheese
1 tablespoon low-fat plain yogurt

1 tablespoon walnuts, chopped
1 teaspoon fresh thyme leaves
Salt and freshly ground black
  pepper

Preheat the oven to 350°F. Combine the mushroom stem with the cheese, yogurt, walnuts, and thyme. Season the mushroom cap and fill with the cheese mixture. Bake for 15 to 20 minutes and serve.

FAST DAY TIP: Goat cheese is lower in calories than cheese made from cow's milk, though this recipe also works well with crumbled Stilton.

... pesto, pine nuts, and ricotta

283 CALORIES PER PORTION

Serves 1

1 large meadow mushroom, cleaned and trimmed, stem removed and chopped
1 scallion, chopped
Zest of ½ lemon
1 teaspoon lemon juice
1 tablespoon pesto sauce

1 tablespoon pine nuts
1¾ ounces/50g ricotta cheese
Salt and freshly ground black pepper
Fresh basil leaves, for serving

Preheat the oven to 350°F. Combine the mushroom stem with the scallion, lemon zest and juice, pesto, pine nuts, and ricotta and mix well. Season the mushroom and spoon the pesto sauce into the cap, then bake in a small roasting pan for 15 to 20 minutes. Serve topped with basil leaves.

OPTIONAL EXTRA: Add a handful of finely chopped rehydrated porcini mushrooms to the pesto sauce for extra earthiness.

THE BEST LENTIL DAHL

203 CALORIES PER PORTION

Serves 6 as a side dish

Cook it long and slow, following each step for the necessary buildup of complex flavors. Find a consistency which suits you—thick, thin, your choice—or add more stock for dahl soup.

10½ ounces/300g chana dahl (yellow dried split peas), rinsed

5 cups/1.2l water

1 vegetable bouillon cube

1 tablespoon sunflower oil

1 tablespoon cumin seeds

1 medium onion, diced

3 green chiles, halved

¾-inch/2cm piece fresh ginger, peeled and julienned

3 garlic cloves, peeled and left whole

3 medium tomatoes, quartered

2 teaspoons ground turmeric

1 teaspoon garam masala

1 teaspoon ground coriander

1 teaspoon lemon juice

Scant ½ cup/100ml water

Salt and freshly ground black pepper

Handful of fresh parsley, chopped, for serving

Place the lentils and water in a pan with the bouillon cube, stir, and bring to a boil. Skim off any froth—be sure to do this or the dahl will be bitter. Cover and reduce the heat. Simmer, stirring regularly, for 35 to 40 minutes, or until the lentils are just tender, adding more water as necessary. Meanwhile, heat the oil in another saucepan over medium heat. Add the cumin seeds and toast for 20 to 30 seconds, then add the onion, chiles, and ginger and sauté for 3 to 4 minutes. Blitz the garlic and tomatoes in a food processor and add the puree to the pan, stirring well to combine. Add the ground spices, lemon juice, and another ½ cup water and stir well. Simmer for 5 minutes, then stir this spiced mix into the cooked lentils, adding more water if necessary. Cook for another 10 minutes. Check the seasoning—you may want to add a little salt once the lentils are cooked through (adding it earlier may make them tough). Serve with plenty of parsley.

WHAT TO DO WITH
A CAN OF BEANS . . .

. . . smashed cannellini with chiles and olives

226 CALORIES PER PORTION

Serves 2 as a side dish

1 (14-ounce/400g) can cannellini
  beans, rinsed and drained
2 garlic cloves, peeled and
  left whole
1 dried chile
1 sprig fresh sage
¼ cup water
Salt and freshly ground black
  pepper

2 teaspoons lemon juice
2 teaspoons olive oil
1 teaspoon red pepper flakes
1¾ ounces/50g small black pitted
  olives
3½ ounces/100g baby spinach
  leaves

Heat the beans, garlic, chile, sage, and water in a saucepan. Season and cook for 3 minutes. Remove the garlic, chile, and sage, then mash the beans coarsely with a fork. Season well. Add the lemon juice, oil, red pepper flakes, olives, and spinach. Stir and serve.

... white beans with pesto

Serves 2 as a side dish

Cooking spray
1 medium onion, finely chopped
1 garlic clove, crushed
1 bay leaf
1 (14-ounce/400g) can cannellini
  beans, rinsed and drained

2 tablespoons pesto sauce
Salt and freshly ground black
  pepper
Lemon wedges and basil leaves,
  for serving

Heat a small frying pan and spray with oil. Sauté the onion, garlic, and bay leaf for 3 minutes on medium heat until softened. Add the beans and heat through. Remove from the heat and add the pesto sauce. Season and stir well to combine. Serve with lemon wedges and a handful of basil leaves.

... big baked beans

265 CALORIES PER PORTION

Serves 2 as a side dish

Cooking spray
1 medium onion, finely chopped
1 (14-ounce/400g) can butter
  beans, rinsed and drained
2 tablespoons tomato paste

½ teaspoon red pepper flakes
1 teaspoon paprika
¾ cup/200g canned diced
  tomatoes
1 teaspoon dried mixed herbs

Heat a pan coated with cooking spray and sauté the onion until softened. Stir in the butter beans, tomato paste, red pepper flakes, paprika, tomatoes, and mixed herbs and simmer for 10 minutes, then serve.

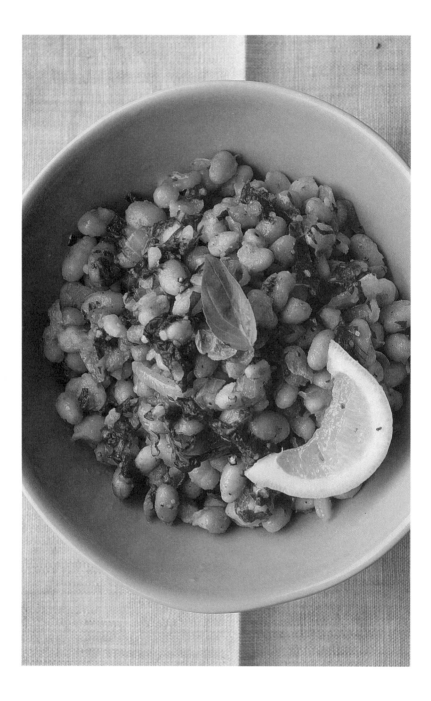

... **sweet and spiced coconut butter beans**

316 CALORIES PER PORTION

Serves 2 as a side dish

2 teaspoons olive oil

1 teaspoon mustard seeds

4 dried curry leaves

1 medium onion, finely chopped

1 tablespoon shredded coconut

1 teaspoon ground turmeric

½ teaspoon ground ginger

1 red chile, seeded and finely sliced

2 medium ripe tomatoes, cored and finely chopped

1 tablespoon mango chutney

Salt and freshly ground black pepper

1 (14-ounce/400g) can butter beans, rinsed and drained

2 teaspoons lemon juice

3½ ounces/100g baby spinach

Heat the oil in a frying pan, add the mustard seeds, and sauté for 1 minute. Add the curry leaves, onion, coconut, turmeric, ginger, and chile and cook until the onion has softened. Add the tomatoes, mango chutney, salt, and pepper and cook for another 3 minutes. Stir in the butter beans with the lemon juice and continue to cook until they are heated through. Remove from the heat and add the spinach leaves. Combine and serve when the spinach has just wilted.

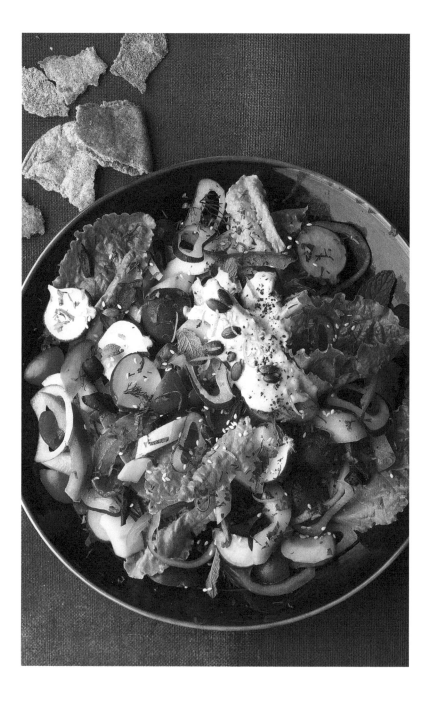

FATOUSH SALAD

242 CALORIES PER PORTION

Serves 4 as a side dish

For the salad
1 large romaine lettuce, coarsely chopped
3 medium ripe tomatoes, coarsely chopped (and peeled if you prefer)
1 medium cucumber, peeled, seeded, and chopped
1 medium red onion, finely sliced
1 medium green bell pepper, seeded and chopped
12 radishes, halved
12 black olives, pitted and chopped
Generous handful of fresh curly parsley, chopped
Small bunch of fresh mint leaves, chopped
Small bunch of fresh dill, chopped
2 whole wheat pitas (6½-inch diameter), toasted and torn into bite-size pieces

For the dressing
2 tablespoons olive oil
1 tablespoon Dijon mustard
2 tablespoons white wine vinegar
1 garlic clove, finely crushed
Salt and cracked black pepper

For the lemon-yogurt sauce
¾ cup/150g low-fat plain yogurt
1 tablespoon tahini
1 tablespoon lemon juice
Zest of ½ lemon
½ teaspoon dried basil
½ teaspoon sumac
Salt and freshly ground black pepper

Handful of chopped herbs and 1 tablespoon seeds for serving (choose from sunflower, sesame, mustard, poppy, pumpkin, or use a mix)

Place the salad ingredients in a large bowl. Prepare dressing by combining all the ingredients and whisking well to emulsify. In a separate bowl, mix the ingredients for the yogurt sauce. Pour the dressing over the salad ingredients, toss well, then drizzle the yogurt sauce on top. Add a scatter of seeds and serve with a final flourish of herbs.

WHAT TO PUT IN A PEPPER . . .

Think of a pepper as a vessel for flavor and texture; the red and yellow varieties tend to be sweeter than the green.

. . . green lentils and porcini

247 CALORIES PER PORTION

Serves 1

Cooking spray
½ medium red onion, diced
1 garlic clove, crushed
2 teaspoons/10g porcini
mushrooms, rehydrated
in boiling water, drained
and chopped, reserving
3 tablespoons/50ml
mushroom water

3½ ounces/100g ready-to-eat
green lentils
Pinch of dried thyme, or
1 teaspoon fresh thyme leaves
1 medium bell pepper, halved
and seeded
1 teaspoon olive oil
Salt and freshly ground black
pepper

Preheat the oven to 350°F. Heat a small pan, lightly spray with oil, and sauté the onion until softened. Add the garlic, stir, and cook for another minute. Add the porcini, stir, and cook for 2 minutes, then add the lentils, thyme, and the mushroom water. Season well and heat through. Place the bell pepper in a small roasting pan, drizzle with a little oil, and bake for 10 minutes. Add the lentil mixture, check the seasoning, and bake for another 10 to 15 minutes.

...feta, tomato, and chickpeas

342 CALORIES PER PORTION

Serves 1

Cooking spray
1 scallion, finely sliced
½ teaspoon paprika
7 ounces/200g canned chickpeas, rinsed and drained
1 medium ripe tomato, chopped
1 tablespoon lemon juice
3 tablespoons/50g feta, crumbled
1 tablespoon chopped fresh flat-leaf parsley
Salt and freshly ground black pepper
1 medium bell pepper, halved and seeded
1 teaspoon olive oil

Preheat the oven to 350°F. Heat a small saucepan, lightly spray with oil, and sauté the scallion until softened. Add the paprika, stir, and cook for another minute. Remove from the heat. Add the chickpeas, tomato, lemon juice, feta, and parsley and season well. Place the bell pepper in a small roasting pan, drizzle with a little oil, and bake for 10 minutes. Add the chickpea mixture and bake for another 10 to 15 minutes.

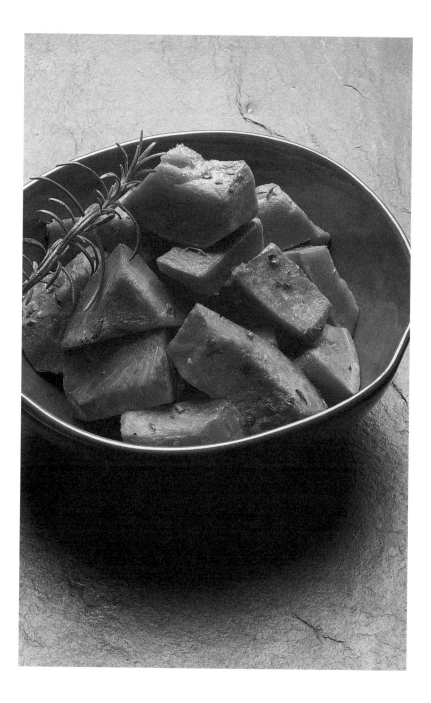

BUTTERNUT SQUASH WITH ROSEMARY AND LIME

260 CALORIES PER PORTION

Serves 2 as a side dish

1 small butternut squash,
peeled, seeded, and cut into
¾-inch/2cm chunks
1 tablespoon olive oil
Juice of 1 lime

2 teaspoons finely chopped fresh
rosemary leaves
Salt and freshly ground black
pepper

Preheat the oven to 350°F. Arrange the butternut in a roasting pan, dress with oil, lime juice, rosemary, salt, and pepper. Bake for 30 minutes, turning once during cooking time.

OPTIONAL EXTRA: Serve with steamed broccoli florets, roasted pumpkin seeds (+60 calories per tablespoon), and a crumble of feta (+25 calories per tablespoon).

● Goes well with Beef and Beer Casserole, page 79 (+398 calories per portion). But since combining these two dishes is over 600 calories, eat a half portion and save the rest.

A HOST OF GOOD THINGS TO SLING ON LEAVES OR GREENS

A simple leaf salad can be transformed into a more interesting and substantial supper with the addition of protein, color, and crunch. Try adding any of the following (all calorie counts are for 3 tablespoons/50g unless otherwise stated).

- bamboo shoots, water chestnuts, and bean sprouts **+15 calories**

- thinly sliced red onion, celery root, or fennel **+15 calories**

- steamed broccoli florets and pickled ginger **+18 calories**

- shredded carrot and zucchini "noodles" **+20 calories**

- edamame **+30 calories**

- 1 tablespoon of pecans or walnuts **+50 calories**

- 1 tablespoon of roasted seeds or pine nuts **+58 calories**

- marinated tofu cubes **+70 calories**

- 6 orange segments **+25 calories** and a tablespoon of hazelnuts **+50 calories**

- hard-boiled egg **+80 calories** per medium egg, or quail's eggs

- 1 fresh fig **+30 calories** and torn low-fat mozzarella **+80 calories**

- homemade oven-dried tomatoes **+125 calories**

- goat cheese **+130 calories** and blueberries (excellent with spinach leaves) **+24 calories**

- cooked chickpeas **+170 calories**

- crumbled Stilton **+150 calories** and pear slices **+50 calories**

THE FAST DAY DRESSING

112 CALORIES PER TABLESPOON

. . . the only one you really need.

1 tablespoon lemon juice
1 tablespoon white wine
vinegar
2 tablespoons olive oil
2 teaspoons Dijon mustard

1 garlic clove, peeled and
left whole
Salt and freshly ground black
pepper

Whisk all the ingredients together and keep in an airtight jar in the fridge. It will last for a week. Remove the garlic clove before eating.

● Try this dressing with flavored vinegars.

FAST DAY TIP: Extra-virgin olive oil is heart-friendly and will give you the best taste in a dressing. Most oils clock up 120 calories per tablespoon, so use sparingly—perhaps just a teaspoon. If you are rationing those Fast Day calories, consider dressing your salad with just a dash of balsamic vinegar. It's only 14 calories per tablespoon.

CILANTRO AND CHILI DIPPING SAUCE

19 CALORIES PER TABLESPOON

3 garlic cloves

1 teaspoon brown sugar

1 teaspoon grated galangal or fresh ginger

½ tablespoon tamarind paste

2 teaspoons lime juice

2 tablespoons water

Fresh cilantro leaves, chopped

2 small red chiles

Blitz all the ingredients in a food processor and serve a spoonful alongside grilled white fish or any simple dish that needs a bolt of fire.

QUICK TOMATO COULIS

26 CALORIES PER PORTION

Serves 6 as a sauce on the side

Less caloric than store-bought sauces, which tend to have hidden sugars and preservatives. Make a batch and freeze in Fast Day portions.

1 (14-ounce/400g) can diced tomatoes

2 tablespoons tomato paste

½ teaspoon honey

Salt and freshly ground black pepper

2 teaspoons dried herb of choice (oregano or mixed herbs)

Put all the ingredients in a small saucepan and simmer for 10 minutes to reduce slightly. Blend for a smoother consistency.

HOMEMADE OVEN-DRIED TOMATOES

20 CALORIES PER 3½ OUNCES/100G

This is one to make in high summer, when tomatoes are at their flavorful best.

20 medium ripe plum tomatoes
Sea salt
6 garlic cloves, crushed
3 tablespoons fresh oregano, chopped

1 tablespoon dried oregano
2 tablespoons extra-virgin olive oil
1 teaspoon sugar
Freshly ground black pepper

Preheat the oven to 250°F. Slice the tomatoes in half and scoop out the seeds. Salt well—a coarse salt works best here—and place, cut side down, on a wire rack or paper towels. Leave for 30 minutes, then rinse and dry. In a small bowl, combine the garlic, oregano, oil, sugar, and pepper and dot the mixture on the tomato halves. Place the tomatoes on a wire rack over a roasting pan and bake for 3 hours, checking occasionally. Cool and store in an airtight container in the fridge. They'll last for 2 to 3 weeks.

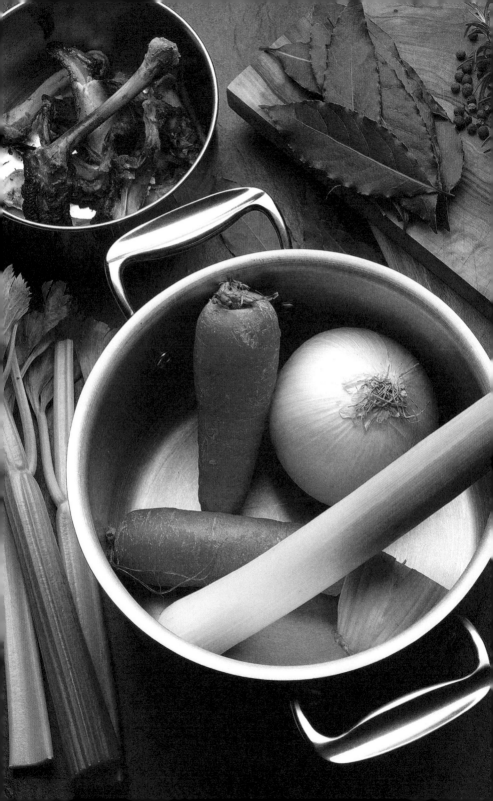

Supper Soups

Warm. And Wise.

Soup is quick to make and brilliantly satiating, an all-around glory that is sometimes overlooked as we reach for a meat-and-two-vegetables meal. A decent stock is essential—without it your soup will almost certainly let you down. What you really need on a Fast Day is an honest, nourishing soup, preferably with some protein in it (beans and lentils will do the trick). For these calorie-controlled soups, I have skimmed off as much fat as possible and turned up the dial on taste.

STOCKY STOCK: THE WORLD'S EASIEST SOUP

VIRTUALLY NIL CALORIES

Have stock handy in the freezer; simply heat it up and add plenty of frozen veggies or herbs and you've got yourself a bowl of Fast Day flavor.

A few stock tips:

● Roasting bones before adding them to the stockpot will boost color and flavor; a roasted chicken carcass is ideal.

● Don't chuck lone bones: freeze them and make a stock when you have a quantity.

● Along with carrot, celery, and onion, add a bouquet garni for herby depth.

● Adding a teaspoon of vinegar to a stock will aid the extraction of minerals without unduly influencing the flavor.

● Don't salt a stock; season the final dish instead to avoid oversalting.

● Once brought to a boil and skimmed, simmer—a good stock should not be rushed or it will turn cloudy.

● Vegetable stock generally has a lower fat content than chicken stock.

● Once strained, be sure to skim off any fat and froth that rises to the top of the pot. Place paper towels on the surface to absorb oils, or chill first to make skimming easier

● If keeping a stock for later use, retain the layer of fat on top to protect it in the fridge. Simply skim when you're ready to use.

● If you are freezing stock, boil the strained stock down in order to reduce it by about half. This will condense the flavor and save freezer space; add water when ready to use.

What to add to the basic stock:

VEGETABLES: sugar snaps, snow peas, broccoli florets, edamame, baby spinach, a handful of herbs, scallions, bamboo shoots, flageolet beans, peas, corn, green beans

PROTEIN: Strips of chicken breast, shrimp, tofu. Or add a handful of dried porcini or cèpes (rehydrate by soaking in boiling water for 30 minutes to make them plump; add the resulting liquor water to the stock for extra oomph); 3½ ounces/100g dried porcini mushrooms has 26 calories and no fat, so they're a great Fast Day standby. Or try "dried mixed forest mushrooms" for more depth.

FLAVOR: If you're not adding fat, you do need to incorporate flavor from elsewhere. Add miso, bouillon cubes, or bouillon powder to capitalize on taste. Then play around with herbs, spices, chiles, fish sauce, lime juice— whatever it takes to make a soup sing.

And to turn it into a satisfying Fast Day soup . . .

● Use clear vegetable stocks. Miso soup and pho, for instance, are lower in calories than dense chowders, bisques, and cream soups.

● Thicken stock with legumes rather than potatoes as they are lower GI. A handful of lentils should be adequate, or a can of cannellini beans, blitzed or mashed once hot.

● Make soup in generous batches and freeze—smooth, thick soups tend to freeze best—and remember that soups, like stews, often taste better the next day.

● When making a soup base, don't sweat onions in butter; use water or a scant spray of oil.

WATERCRESS AND ZUCCHINI SOUP WITH PARMESAN AND PINE NUTS

126 CALORIES PER PORTION

Serves 4

1 tablespoon olive oil
1 large onion, diced
1 pound/450g zucchini,
  chopped
1¾ ounces/50g potatoes, peeled
  and chopped
1 garlic clove, crushed
5¼ cups/1.25l vegetable stock

9 ounces/200g watercress,
  thicker stems removed
1 tablespoon pine nuts
Salt and freshly ground black
  pepper
1 tablespoon grated Parmesan
  cheese
Fresh basil leaves

Heat the oil in a large pan, add the onion, and sauté till softened but not browned. Add the zucchini, potatoes, and garlic, sweat for 10 minutes, then add the stock. Simmer for another 10 minutes, partially covered, adding watercress for the final 3 minutes. Meanwhile, toast the pine nuts and set aside. Blitz the soup with a hand blender, adjust the consistency by adding extra water or stock if necessary, and season. Reheat and serve with a scatter of Parmesan, pine nuts, and basil leaves.

OPTIONAL EXTRA: Serve topped with a soft poached egg instead of Parmesan and pine nuts.

EGG-DROP SOUP

161 CALORIES PER PORTION

Serves 2

This soup is simplicity itself, but it does rely on a decent stock, so go for the best you can get—either homemade or store-bought in a carton.

5 cups/1.2l good, flavorful chicken stock, skimmed of fat
2 large eggs
Salt and freshly ground black pepper

2 or 3 scallions, finely chopped
Small bunch of fresh flat-leaf parsley, coarsely chopped

Heat the stock until just simmering. Whisk the eggs in a small bowl, season with a pinch of salt and pepper, add 1 tablespoon water, and then pour in a slow, thin stream into the simmering stock, stirring as you go to create elegant silken strands. Serve immediately, topped with a scatter of scallions and parsley. For an Italian take on egg-drop soup, make stracciatella by adding 1 tablespoon grated Parmesan, 1 teaspoon lemon zest, 1 teaspoon freshly chopped marjoram, and a little nutmeg to the egg mix before the drop (add 20 calories for the Parmesan).

OPTIONAL EXTRA: Add a handful or two of frozen peas and some baby spinach leaves to the hot stock, then bring back to a simmer before adding the egg.

TOM YUM

Serves 2

5 cups/1.2l good chicken or vegetable stock
1 teaspoon shrimp paste
1 lemongrass stalk, smashed
2 kaffir lime leaves
¾-inch/2cm piece fresh ginger or galangal, peeled and sliced
Small handful of fresh cilantro, including stalks, chopped
1 chile, halved and seeded
5 ounces/150g raw jumbo shrimp or squid rings (fresh or frozen)
2 scallions, finely sliced on the diagonal

Handful of bok choy, sliced
3½ ounces/100g green beans, blanched
10 cherry tomatoes, halved
1 tablespoon mirin
1 tablespoon Thai fish sauce
1 tablespoon soy sauce
1 tablespoon lime juice
½ teaspoon palm sugar or light muscovado sugar
Fresh cilantro leaves, red chile, and lime zest, for serving

In a large pan, heat the stock, shrimp paste, lemongrass, lime leaves, ginger, cilantro, and chile. Simmer for 15 minutes then strain and return the clear stock to the pan. Reheat and add the shrimp, together with the scallions. Simmer for another 3 minutes. Add the bok choy, green beans, tomatoes, mirin, fish sauce, soy sauce, lime juice, and sugar. Continue to simmer for 2 to 3 minutes, or until the vegetables are just tender. Serve sprinkled with cilantro leaves, a little more red chile, and a grating of lime zest.

● This also works well with 5 ounces/150g chicken breast fillet, cut into thin strips and added to the hot stock.

OPTIONAL EXTRA: Try adding some shiitake mushrooms, bamboo shoots, silken tofu, or edamame.

EASY PEA AND HAM

228 CALORIES PER PORTION

Serves 4

1 teaspoon butter
4¼ cups/1l ham or chicken stock,
 skimmed of fat
1 medium onion, diced
1 medium potato, peeled
 and diced

1 ham or chicken bouillon cube
1 pound/450g frozen baby peas
7 ounces/200g thick sliced ham,
 trimmed of any fat and diced
Salt and freshly ground black
 pepper

Heat the butter and 2 tablespoons of the stock in a saucepan and gently sweat the onion until translucent. Add the potato, the remaining stock and the bouillon cube, and simmer for 10 minutes. Add the peas and bring back to a simmer for 2 to 3 minutes. Remove from the heat and blitz with a hand blender until smooth. Stir in the diced ham, adjust the seasoning if necessary (the bouillon cube and ham may make the soup salty enough already). Serve, perhaps in a mug, on a cold day.

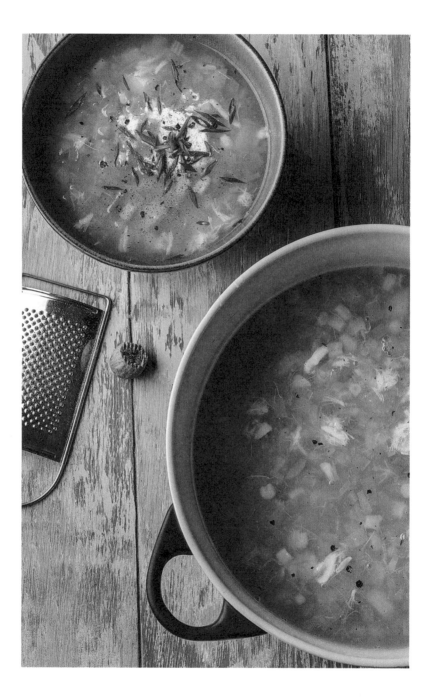

CRAB AND CORN CHOWDER

248 CALORIES PER PORTION

Serves 4

1 medium onion, finely diced

1 medium leek, trimmed and finely chopped

2 medium celery stalks, finely chopped

2 medium carrots, peeled and finely chopped

4¼ cups/1l chicken or vegetable stock

2 medium potatoes, peeled and diced

7 ounces/200g frozen corn

6 ounces/170g can white crabmeat, drained

3 tablespoons low-fat crème fraîche

Salt and freshly ground black pepper

Snipped chives and freshly grated nutmeg, for serving

Place the onion, leek, celery, and carrots in a large saucepan and add a few tablespoons of the stock. Sweat over medium heat for about 10 minutes, stirring regularly until soft and taking care that they don't stick (add a dash more stock if it threatens to). Add the potatoes and the remaining stock, stir, and simmer for 10 to 15 minutes, or until the potato is tender. Add the corn and crabmeat, then simmer for another 3 minutes. Remove from the heat, stir in the crème fraîche, and season well with salt and plenty of pepper. Serve with a scatter of chives and nutmeg.

OPTIONAL EXTRA: For a deeper, richer flavor, add 3½ ounces/100g diced pancetta to the onions as they sauté (+100 calories per portion). Or make a curried version by adding 2 teaspoons curry powder along with the potatoes.

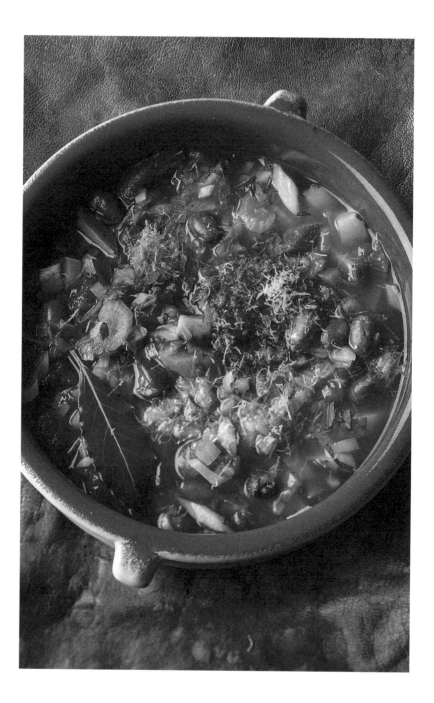

PISTOU

284 CALORIES FOR THE STOCK + 117 FOR THE PISTOU

Serves 2

Pistou is a Provençal sauce made from garlic and basil. The Argentines make a similar sauce called chimichurri, which relies on parsley and chile. But the point of these—and of pesto—is the same: a whack of flavor. Here, pistou wakes up a good veggie stock. But you could just as well serve it alongside plain grilled chicken or steak.

For the stock
Cooking spray
1 medium onion, finely diced
1 large leek, trimmed and finely sliced
1 medium fennel bulb, finely chopped
2 medium carrots, peeled and finely chopped
2 medium zucchini, finely chopped
1 bay leaf
1 medium celery stalk, finely chopped
1 tablespoon chopped fresh flat-leaf parsley
1 (14-ounce/400g) can cannellini beans, rinsed and drained

1 (14-ounce/400g) can diced tomatoes
2 cups/500ml chicken or vegetable stock
Salt and freshly ground black pepper
Lemon zest, for serving

For the pistou sauce
3 garlic cloves
Small handful of fresh basil leaves
2 tablespoons olive oil
2 ounces/60g Parmesan cheese, grated
½ teaspoon sea salt

Spray a large saucepan with oil and sauté the onion and leek for 3 to 4 minutes over medium heat, stirring and adding a spoonful or two of stock if they stick. Add all the other stock ingredients to the pan, stir, season lightly, and simmer until the vegetables are tender, about 15 minutes. For the pistou sauce, put the ingredients in a blender and pulse to a smooth paste. Serve the hot soup in a deep bowl with a dollop of pistou and a final grating of lemon zest.

BUTTERNUT SQUASH SOUP WITH SPICED SAFFRON YOGURT

285 CALORIES PER PORTION

Serves 4

2¼ pounds/1kg butternut squash, peeled, seeded, and chopped
1 pound/450g tomatoes, quartered and cored (and peeled if you wish)
2 garlic cloves, peeled
2 medium carrots, peeled and chopped
1 medium onion, chopped
1 tablespoon olive oil
1 teaspoon red pepper flakes
2 star anise
2 teaspoons ground cumin
2 teaspoons ground coriander
2 teaspoons paprika

1½ quarts/1.5l vegetable stock
3½ ounces/100g red lentils
Salt and freshly ground black pepper

For the saffron yogurt
¾ cup/150g low-fat plain yogurt
Small pinch of saffron threads
1 teaspoon cumin seeds
1 teaspoon ground cumin

Generous pinch of fresh sage leaves and 1 tablespoon toasted pumpkin seeds (optional), for serving

Preheat the oven to 350°F. Place the butternut squash, tomatoes, garlic, carrots, and onion in a roasting pan and drizzle with oil. Add the spices and mix well, then cover with foil and bake until everything is tender, about an hour. Remove the star anise from the pan. In a large saucepan, coarsely mash the baked vegetables and stir in the stock. Bring to a simmer, then add the lentils and cook on low heat for 20 minutes. Season with salt and pepper, adding a little extra stock if the soup is too thick. If you prefer a smoother soup, blitz with a hand blender; for supreme silkiness, you could even strain it and reheat. Combine the saffron, cumin seeds, and ground cumin in a bowl, stirring well to release the saffron's golden color. Serve the soup in deep bowls with a swirled spoonful of saffron yogurt, a handful of toasted pumpkin seeds (+75 calories per tablespoon), and young sage leaves scattered on top.

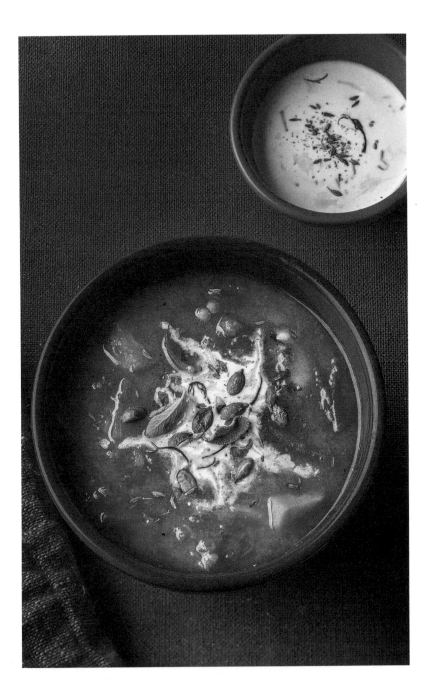

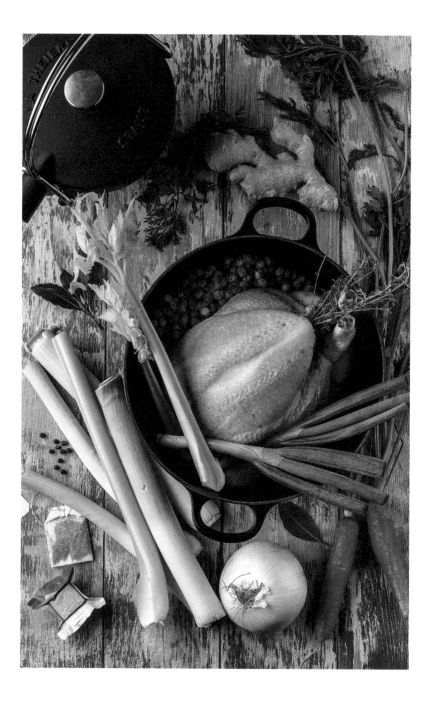

GREEN TEA CHICKEN SOUP

377 CALORIES PER PORTION

Serves 4

The addition of green tea gives this pretty soup a subtle new flavor—
expect delicate rather than bold. By all means, use ready-made
stock and fresh chicken breast rather than cooking the bird whole to
produce a fresh stock.

1 small chicken, washed and
dried (about 2½ pounds/1.2kg)

3 large leeks, trimmed and
coarsely chopped

4 medium carrots, peeled and
chopped

1 medium onion, diced

3 medium celery stalks, chopped

1¼-inch/3cm piece fresh ginger,
peeled and sliced

3 sprigs fresh thyme

1 teaspoon peppercorns

2 bay leaves

1 chicken bouillon cube

1¼ cups/300ml strong green tea,
strained if loose leaf, or tea
bag removed

3½ ounces/100g frozen
baby peas

2 scallions, finely sliced

Juice of 1 lemon

Salt and freshly ground black
pepper

2 tablespoons chopped fresh
curly parsley, for serving

Place the chicken in a large saucepan with the leeks, carrots, onion,
celery, and ginger. Add the thyme, peppercorns, and bay leaves, then
fill the pan with enough cold water to just cover the chicken. Bring to a
boil, then cover and simmer for 1½ hours. Remove the chicken from the
pan, set aside, and strain the stock, skimming off any froth or fat. Return
the stock to the heat and add the crumbled bouillon cube. Meanwhile,
discard the chicken skin and remove the meat from the bones; shred and
return to the pan of stock, along with the green tea, peas, and scallions.
Heat through for 3 to 4 minutes, then add the lemon juice and season
well. Serve sprinkled with parsley—don't omit this, it's part of the delicate
charm of the dish.

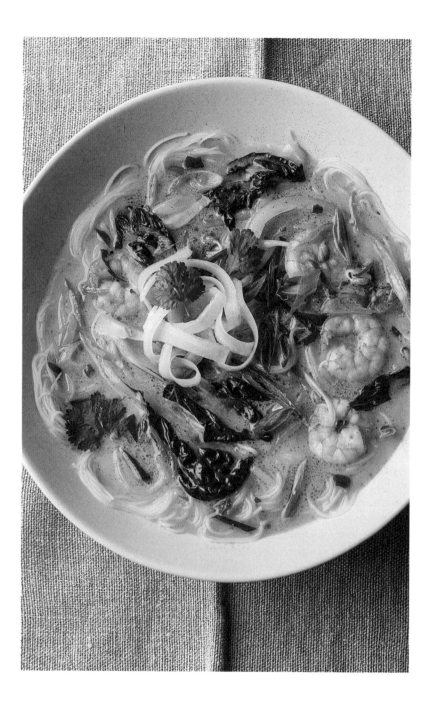

SHRIMP LAKSA

400 CALORIES PER PORTION

Serves 2

This spiced Malaysian noodle soup is a proper meal in a bowl and has a fairly generous number of calories to match (but it's worth every last one of them).

5¼ ounces/150g fine rice noodles
2 tablespoons laksa paste
 from a jar
1¾ cups/400ml low-fat
 coconut milk
2 cups/500ml chicken stock
3 scallions, finely sliced on
 the diagonal, a few slices
 reserved for garnish

1 red chile, halved, seeded, and
 finely sliced
3½ ounces/100g shrimp, fresh or
 cooked
3½ ounces/100g bean sprouts
1 bok choy, thinly sliced
¼ medium cucumber, peeled,
 seeded, and cut into fine strips
 lengthwise, and a handful of
 fresh cilantro leaves, for serving

Prepare the noodles according to the package directions and set aside. Heat a large saucepan, add the laksa paste and 1 tablespoon of the coconut milk. Sauté for 3 minutes to release the paste's flavor, then add the remaining coconut milk, stock, scallions, and chile. Stir and simmer for 2 minutes. Add the shrimp, bean sprouts, and bok choy and simmer for another 3 minutes, until the shrimp and vegetables are just cooked. Check the seasoning. Place the prepared noodles in bowls and cover with the hot soup. Garnish with delicate strips of cucumber, a little more scallion, and cilantro leaves.

RECIPES BY CALORIE COUNT

Calories	Recipe	Page
0 (virtually)	Stocky Stock	148
15	Bamboo Shoots, Water Chestnuts, and Bean Sprouts (1¾ ounces/50g)	142
	Sliced Red Onion, Celery Root or Fennel (1¾ ounces/50g)	142
18	Steamed Broccoli Florets (1¾ Ounces/50g) and Pickled Ginger	142
19	Cilantro and Chili Dipping Sauce	144
20	Homemade Oven-Dried Tomatoes	145
	Shredded Carrot and Zucchini "Noodles" (1¾ ounces/50g)	142
25	Saffron and Shallot Sauce	67
26	Quick Tomato Coulis	144
27	Spring Greens with Mustard Seeds	111
30	Edamame (1¾ ounces/50g)	142
35	Veggie "Noodles" (3½ ounces/100g)	17
36	Cauliflower "Couscous"	112
50	Tablespoon of Pecans or Walnuts	142
58	Tablespoon of Roasted Seeds or Pine Nuts	142
64	Lemon-Pepper Broccoli with Coconut Oil	113
68	Saag on the Side	26
70	Marinated Tofu Cubes (1¾ ounces/50g)	142
74	Chunky Cumin Coleslaw	114
75	6 Orange Segments and a Tablespoon of Hazelnuts	142
79	Spiced Red Cabbage with Apples	115
80	Hard-Boiled Egg	142
92	Celery Root Remoulade	116
105	Shrimp and Asparagus Stir-Fry	36
110	Fresh Fig and (1¾ ounces/50g) Torn Low-Fat Mozzarella	142
112	The Fast Day Dressing	143
123	Baked Fennel with Parmesan and Thyme	119
	Tabbouleh	117
124	Chunky Cumin Coleslaw	114
125	Homemade Oven-Dried Tomatoes 1¾ ounces/50g	145

Calories	Recipe	Page
126	Watercress and Zucchini Soup with Parmesan and Pine Nuts	150
133	Asian Sesame Salad	121
140	Chicken, Gremolata, and Dark Leaves	38
142	Cauliflower Mash	122
144	Mexican Black Bean Chili	13
150-190	Fast Day Plain Omelet	56
150-465	Fast Day Omelet Variations	56
154	Goat Cheese (1¾ ounces/50g) and Blueberries (1¾ ounces/50g)	142
154	Stuffed Pepper with Green Lentils and Porcini	138
161	Egg-Drop Soup	151
162	Chicken Tagine with Preserved Lemons and Saffron	64
170	Cooked Chickpeas (1¾ ounces/50g)	142
171	Spiced Brown Lentils with Mint Salad	124
173	Stuffed Mushroom with Spinach, Chile, and Cheese	128
173	Tom Yum	152
173	Turkey Kofte with Tzatziki (No Pita)	100
175	No-Fuss Fish with Chili Dressing	45
179	Chicken, Peppers, and Capers	41
179	Neapolitan Cianfotta (Summer Vegetable Stew)	68
180	Bean Bolognese	18
180	Skinny Spaghetti Bolognese	17
183	Cannellini Bean Mash	122
183	Simple Seared Sirloin	86
183	Sweet Potato and Carrot Mash	123
200	Crumbled Stilton (1¾ ounces/50g) and Pear Slices (1¾ ounces/50g)	142
203	The Best Lentil Dahl	131
207	One-Pot Bean Feast	70
210	Dijon Marinated Chicken	42
219	Mexican Black Bean Chili with Avocado	13
215	Garlic and Parsley Shrimp	91
220	Bean Bolognese with Olives	18
220	Cod Arrabbiata	63

Calories	Recipe	Page
221	Chicken Masala and Raita	43
222	Ten-Minute Jumbo Shrimp Curry	92
226	Smashed Cannellini with Chile and Olives	132
228	Easy Pea and Ham Soup	153
230	Beef Chili Stir-Fry	93
234	Lamb Burgers with Hot Tomato Sauce	94
239	Coq au Vin	20
241	Low-Cal Chili Con Carne	15
242	Fatoush Salad	137
247	Fire and Spice Veggie Casserole	71
247	Stuffed Pepper with Green Lentils and Porcini	138
248	Crab and Corn Chowder	155
248	Five-Minute Roast Beef Salad	49
249	Chickpea Curry in a Hurry	50
253	Yellow Squash and Almond Salad	125
254	White Beans with Pesto	133
260	Butternut Squash with Rosemary and Lime	141
262	Three-Pepper Fajita Salad	101
263	Lamb Chops with Peas	95
263	Sirloin Steak, Arugula, and Watercress with Horseradish Cream	86
263	Tex-Mex Chicken	40
264	Chicken and Cabbage Chop Suey	62
265	Big Baked Beans	133
267	Easy Lamb Kebabs	97
273	Buffalo Chicken Burgers with Blue Cheese and Celery Relish	106
273	Chinese Spiced Chicken	44
275	Hot Paprika Goulash	23
275	Stuffed Mushroom with Goat Cheese and Walnut	129
276	Smoked Salmon Gratin	25
278	Yellow Squash and Almond Salad with Feta	125
279	Tandoori Chicken with Mint Dip and Saag on the Side	26
283	Huevos Rancheros	98
283	Stuffed Mushroom with Pesto, Pine Nut, and Ricotta	130

Calories	Recipe	Page
284	Chickpea Curry in a Hurry with Spinach or Tomatoes	50
285	Butternut Squash Soup with Saffron Yogurt	158
287	Chipotle-Glazed Individual Meat Loaves	18
	Sirloin Steak with Pepper Sauce	87
290	Fish Tacos	51
292	Sirloin Steak with Chili Dipping Sauce and Bok Choy	87
293	Chicken Salsa Verde	78
	Roast Beef Hash with Eggs	32
294	Basic Boeuf Bourguignon	27
299	Pork Milanese with Arugula	46
302	White Chili with Turkey	14
310	Turkey Kofte with Tzatziki and Warm Pita	100
311	Vegetable Tagine with Herbed Couscous	65
313	Sirloin Steak with Herb Dressing	88
316	Sweet and Spiced Coconut Butter Beans	135
318	Chicken Cassoulet	73
319	Chickpea Curry in a Hurry with Almonds	50
323	Sirloin Steak with Baked Tomatoes and Olives	88
328	Italian Rabbit Stew	75
331	Super-Fast Thai Green Chicken Curry	28
335	Panko "Fried" Chicken	103
337	Fast Day Biryani	29
340	Cottage Pie	30
342	Stuffed Pepper with Feta, Tomato, and Chickpea	139
348	Chicken Provençal	76
	Crab and Corn Chowder with Pancetta	155
349	Moroccan Spiced Lamb Tagine	67
358	Green Lentil, Orange, and Hazelnut Salad	126
360	Beef Chili Stir-Fry with Fresh Egg Noodles	93
365	Smoked Salmon and Shrimp Gratin	33
370	Butternut Squash with Rosemary, Lime, Broccoli, Pumpkin Seeds, and Feta	141
	Chicken Sausage Jambalaya	77

Calories	Recipe	Page
377	Green Tea Chicken Soup	161
385	Sea Bass with Tomato, Chorizo, and Butter Beans	105
386	Quick Roast Pork Loin with Broccoli, Cauliflower, and Cheese Sauce	52
390	Moussaka	31
398	Beef and Beer Casserole	79
400	Shrimp Laksa	163
401	Boston Beans and Ham	80
401	Pistou and Stock	157
415	Sea Bass with Tomato, Chorizo, Butter Beans, and Olives	105
418	Green Lentil, Orange, and Hazelnut Salad with Tofu	126
429	Beef Daube with Peppered Greens	82
467	Peppered Pork with Summer Slaw	54
493	Peppered Pork with Warm Winter Slaw	55
548	Huevos Rancheros with Avocado, Chili Sauce, and Tortilla	98

ACKNOWLEDGMENTS

Little did we know, when we first gathered at the Clerkenwell Kitchen on a chilly October day in 2012, that *The FastDiet* would cause such an almighty stir. My thanks, heartfelt and constant, go to Aurea Carpenter and Rebecca Nicolson of Short Books, and to the ever-brilliant team at Atria: Judith Curr, Sarah Durand, Benjamin Lee, Paul Olsewski, Lisa Sciambra, Jeanne Lee, Daniella Wexler, Kimberly Goldstein, Kristen Lemire, Dana Sloan, and Stacey Kulig. And, of course, to Dr. Michael Mosley, who responded to the 3 a.m. text message that launched a diet phenomenon and changed the lives (and weight) of thousands.

I am ever grateful to Team FastDiet: to Paul Bougourd, Emmie Francis, Klara Zak, and Catherine Gibbs for their ceaseless energy, industry, and support; to Georgia Vaux for her brilliant FastDiet design; and to Annie Hudson, who watched over my recipes and made sure that they didn't stick or burn or contain too much chile (I like it hot). Romas Foord's photos continue to make Fast food look fabulous. And I thank Nicola Jeal, again, because I'll never quite manage to say it enough.

A big thank-you to my mum, Marmalade, fount of culinary wisdom, for her help with *FastDay Cookbook*. And finally, love ever to my sticky-fingered kids—Lily and Ned—and to PBQC. Now that he's on the *FastDiet* too, he keeps telling me how many calories are in a biscuit. Which is, ya'know, quite annoying. . .

INDEX

Join the Diet and Fitness Revolution!

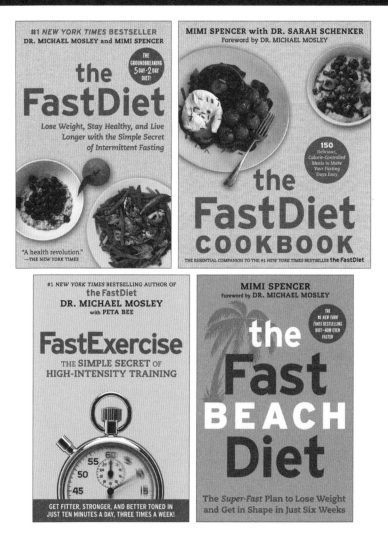

PROUDLY PUBLISHED BY ATRIA BOOKS

Pick up or download your copy today.